The Human Being

Understanding and treatment of the person

by

Dr W Norman Taylor

Augur Press

THE HUMAN BEING:
UNDERSTANDING AND TREATMENT OF THE PERSON

Copyright © Mirabelle Maslin 2014

The moral right of the author has been asserted

Dr W Norman Taylor is also the author of:

Poems of Wartime Years

British Library Cataloguing in Publication Data.
A catalogue record for this book is available from
the British Library.

ISBN 978-0-9571380-3-2
First published 2014 by
Augur Press
Delf House
52 Penicuik Road
Roslin
Midlothian EH25 9LH
United Kingdom

Printed by Lightning Source

The Human Being

Understanding and treatment of the person

Preface

Although I had met Dr Taylor on a number of occasions over a period of years, I did not know him particularly well until the late 1980s. Since that time, he and I often worked very closely together. I found that his drive to understand what troubled a person was almost inexhaustible.

About ten years ago, he gave me the essays and lectures that appear in this book, and I published one of them – *What is Going Wrong?* – in *Carl and other writings*, which is a book I wrote on the subject of sexual abuse of children.

Since Dr Taylor's death in July 2013, I have come to think that I should make this collection of his writings available to others, and I began to prepare them for publication.

From this material any reader will see how closely psychiatry, psychology, psychotherapy and psychoanalysis are interlinked, and how the relatively modern profession of counselling can play an important part in the development of human potential.

Mirabelle Maslin

Contents

Introduction

Dr W Norman Taylor was born in Armadale, West Lothian, in January 1919. He studied medicine at the University of Edinburgh. Throughout his life he demonstrated a wide range of interests, which included literature, poetry and painting, and also the study of languages. He loved hill walking, and climbed many of the Scottish mountains, taking up ice climbing in his 50s. He died in July 2013.

Relatively few of his writings have survived. This book contains several lectures and essays. There is a book of poems – *Poems of Wartime Years* – which was published in 2007. More poems exist, but are as yet unpublished.

As a psychiatrist in the NHS, Dr Taylor's special field became that of psychotherapy (individuals, couples and groups), having a particular interest in marital work with couples. As a university lecturer, he was involved in the training of junior psychiatrists, and also in the training and supervision of nurses, social workers and other professionals, e.g. clergy. He was attached to the Edinburgh University Student Counselling Service for some years. He supervised counsellors in the Edinburgh Marriage Guidance Council for more than 10 years, and for 3 years was its chairman. On retirement from the NHS, he remained a psychotherapist, working privately at the Scottish Institute of Human Relations.

Some fragments of Dr Taylor's writings about the early years of his working life.

I was a medical student when the war began in 1939. I knew that when I qualified I would be called up. I did a short stint as a GP in Fife before being sent to serve with an infantry battalion in coastal defence on the Isle of Wight. After this I was posted to a West African division and accompanied its men into the jungles of Burma. This involved a fight against disease as well as against the Japanese. When this was over, I sailed off with my African soldiers and returned them to their homes in the Gold Coast, now called Ghana.

I was not demobilised until 1946, and before that I served for a short time in a prisoner-of-war camp in Scotland, attending to German prisoners who had come back from Russia. One of them was a doctor, although of course he did not have any kind of official position. He could translate for me the men's medical complaints. The predominant medical conditions I had to deal with were the after-effects of frostbite.

Once back in Edinburgh, I obtained a job with a Hospital Board as a trainee psychiatrist. There was not yet an NHS. I saw many patients who had been incarcerated for years and were totally institutionalised. They included some whose brains had been irreversibly damaged by the 1918 flu epidemic. I became familiar with insulin coma therapy, ECT, deep sedation and the new treatment of leucotomy.

Schizophrenia of its various types was looked upon as an incurable disease, and there was no definitive treatment for it. Dementia praecox was the old term for schizophrenia, which often started in young people. The prognosis for betterment of these conditions was virtually nil, and therefore the patients and their relatives were often not given the true diagnosis. The kind of stigma it carried was terrible.

I saw very little of tertiary syphilis, which used to be called GPI – General Paralysis of the Insane – ultimately fatal.

The introduction of largactil in the early 1950s as a treatment for psychosis, and tofranil for depressive states, revolutionised treatment options. I remember that some were trying LSD as a treatment to see if it worked, but any beneficial effect was patchy and unreliable, and its use was abandoned. I myself had a strong belief in the value of understanding with each patient what was going on in his or her mind. However, I found that I had to be cautious, as I could find that my own sense of reality ran the risk of becoming distorted!

Bowlby's Contribution to the Theory of Personality Development

This paper is based on notes of a lecture to the postgraduate MPhil course at Edinburgh University Department of Psychiatry, 1975. It is an introduction to the work of John Bowlby's revision of psychodynamic theory of personality development and structure. This remit excludes the topic of 'loss', i.e. bereavement and depression, for which he is well known.

Bowlby is a psychoanalyst who was much influenced by the students of animal behaviour – the ethologists, such as Konrad Lorenz and Robert Hinde. To him, ethology was a way of attempting reconciliation between traditional psychodynamic theory and the sciences of zoology and developmental biology.

I thought that it might be interesting to look at
  (a) his basic ideas and methodology
  (b) his views on personal bonding and attachment
  (c) his views on separation and deprivation
  (d) his theories about fear, phobias and 'anxious attachment'
  (e) and finally, some consequences in certain forms of disturbed family interaction and psychopathology.

It is sometimes difficult to remember that he is a psychoanalyst!
  He devotes a great deal of attention to empirical *observation* of children in relation to the family (and the non-family), drawing on studies by the Robertsons, Schaffer, *et al*, as well as his own – unlike some psychoanalytical theorists, who seem to 'deduce' children from the study of neurotic adults. Hence Bowlby's

5

method is ethological: the direct observation of natural behaviour. And the dynamic behind everything is *biological adaptation*, not 'instinctual gratification'. Among other things, it is interesting to note that this view tends to blur the boundaries between so-called 'normal' and 'neurotic' behaviour. On his own admission, his writings miss out all analogies, or even references, to the 'thermodynamic' concept of psychic energy assumed by Freud, who never escaped from the models of 19th century physics. And while he draws a lot from the object-relations psychology of Klein, Winnicott, Balint and Fairbairn, his concept of 'instinct' owes really nothing to psychoanalysis. Central to it is the science of behavioural systems-theory and information processing, the paradigm of 20th century genetics and computer science. He sees so-called 'instinctive' behaviour as a system of integrated and controlled responses, triggered by sensory information, carried through by cybernetic guidance systems, and terminated by distinct consummatory stimuli. No 'psychic energy' peculiar to instinct (what Freud called 'libido') is postulated – only the ordinary physico-chemical energies of physiology. With these concepts Bowlby approaches the problems of personality development by evolving his attachment theory.

Probably nobody doubts that within its first year the infant has developed a strong affectional tie to its mother, or mother figure, in normal circumstances. Bowlby reviewed and analysed the work already done in this field, and distilled it down into four basic alternative theories, viewing them with his ethological eye. He translates the language of 'ego' and 'object' into a less abstract form more compatible with an infant's observed behaviour, and then reduced the traditional theories into the following elemental constituents:

(1) The Theory of Secondary Drive
    This is the original Freudian 'cupboard-love' model. The
    child's attachment to mother is *secondary* to his learning

6

that she satisfies his bodily needs. These primary, in-built needs are physiological: food, warmth, gratification, etc., and are not social.

(2) <u>The Theory of Primary Object-sucking</u>
This is the basic principle in the work of Melanie Klein, Erikson, Sullivan and Spitz, who stress the concept of 'orality' – the primary instinct to suck a breast: 'incorporate the object'.

(3) <u>The Theory of Primary Object-clinging</u>
This is the earliest active seeking-of-mother object-relation, related to security needs rather than libido. It is implied in the work of Alice and Michael Balint (from Hermann the zoologist, who described an 'instinct to cling' in 1936).

(4) <u>The Theory of Return-to-Womb Craving</u>
This is invoked by Klein, Ferenczi and early Fairbairn.

The Secondary Drive and Return-to-Womb theories are considered biologically inadequate, and improbable to say the least, and Bowlby links primary Object-clinging with the related behaviour of Object-following. Both these behaviour patterns are primary forms long since known to ethologists studying birds and mammals, e.g. Lorenz and Hinde. They have the obvious effect of tying an infant to mother, or a similarly related adult, in a way which is *independent of physiological need*. I.e. they promote a tie which is primarily social: a 'social bonding' (see Lorenz's description of imprinting in birds – a social instinct).

This is the essence of Bowlby's ethological model of attachment. 'Attachment', in his technical sense, is behaviour that has the effect of attaining or retaining proximity to some other differentiated and preferred individual. He originally described five primary instinctive behaviour patterns in human infants in the important paper 'The Nature of the Child's Tie to Mother' (Int. J. Psychoanal., 39, 1958), viz, Sucking, Clinging, Following, Smiling and Crying. 'Sucking' appears related to clinging initially, and these two operate at close range. 'Following' (apart from eye following) requires locomotion, while 'crying' and 'smiling' operate at a distance, by stimulating mother to follow and cling.

Together these forms make up the child's Attachment Behaviour.

To understand how this develops we have to consider first the perceptual and cognitive aspects of the child's tie, which are fundamental, in that the activation and termination of behaviour responses depend upon *awareness of the object, as separate from self.* (See H R Schaffer, 'Some Issues for Research in the Study of Attachment Behaviour', p179 of 'Determinants of Infant Behaviour', Ed. Foss.)

In the state at birth, it is presumed that there is no awareness of subject-object difference. Thereafter, as the concept of externality develops, a relation to 'part-objects' precedes the conception of a separate whole person. Alice Balint, Melanie Klein, Winnicott and Spitz have been specially concerned with these problems. Spitz, working on the smile response, distinguished an early phase where the perceived object is *conceptualised* as an external agent, capable of anticipating needs, and belonging in a world of permanently-existing objects outside the self (6 to 9 months). Between these, there is an intermediate stage where, although all the baby reacts to may be a signal rather than a person, his responses become appropriate and discriminating – what Spitz called 'une relation pre-objectale', at 3 to 6 months: a precursor of true object-relation. An authority in this field is Jean Piaget, with his detailed studies of cognitive development.

Transition from the early reaction-to-signals in the here-and-now to being in the world of interacting objects (including himself) in space and time, takes the first 9 months of life. But before that, at about 28 weeks, there is an important intermediate

8

phase, described by Spitz ('Eighth Month Anxiety: A Genetic Field Theory of Ego Formation' – 1959). He points out that after this critical period infants respond differently to familiar and unfamiliar persons, turning towards the former and away from the latter, showing pleasure and displeasure respectively. This accords with the movement from pre-objectal relation to true object-relation. Schaffer noted that children who lose their mothers after this point 'fret', but before it they react differently. The point seems especially critical regarding the conflicts of ambivalence. It probably marks the time when the infant first experiences *both* his rudimentary relationships with 'good-mother-to-be-loved' and 'bad-mother-to-be-hated', linking them both in his mind in conformity with the single, external object – the 'fusion of good relation and bad relation' described by Spitz. Now the fragments of part-objects begin to unite in one and the same source, and there is subsequent recognition that the source is a whole object, existing and operating independently of the self. At this 'sensitive' point, the child's attachment is seen to be discriminatingly to the mother, and consequently *separation from her becomes conceivable* – hence the term 'eighth month anxiety'.

Bowlby undertakes a long and erudite discussion of so-called instinctive behaviour in humans and animals in Volume 1 of his trilogy 'Attachment and Loss'. The psychiatric kernel of this is more succinctly given in 'The Child's Tie to Mother'. He avoids the pitfalls of teleology in discussing the 'aims' of instinct, which he strictly differentiates from the actual causes, quoting the ethological view that their presumed 'aims' (of self and race preservation) are tautological, unnecessary to explain their existence. You don't need to invent an 'instinct to see' in order to explain the existence of the eye! 'Instinctive behaviour' is mediated by cybernetically controlled systems serving the sort of biological adaptation required by a particular organism, at a particular developmental stage, in its familiar environment. These controlled behaviour systems range from simple approach-avoidance to highly complex configurations requiring elaborate programming and intermediate set goals. In biological systems, a structure of this kind takes a form determined not only by inbuilt genetic mechanisms, but also equally by the kind of environment in which the system (or sub-system) has already been operating during its evolution, and in which it will presumably continue to live: its 'environment of evolutionary adaptedness' (Hartmann).

Instinctive behaviour in Bowlby's model is moreover specifically <u>activated</u> and <u>terminated</u> by appropriate stimuli from the object of the behaviour. 'Activation' also requires certain internal conditions, such as hormonal levels, with feelings, thoughts and so on, that conduce to a responsive mood, and perhaps even to 'seeking' behaviour. These enhance responsiveness to the external stimuli. The latter act as the 'releasers' that set off the instinctive response towards the object: they are the trigger signs of Spitz and Piaget. 'Termination' likewise is triggered by specific conditions and signals. Instinctive behaviour does not simply expend itself like kinetic energy according to the principles of thermodynamics, any more than a car stops at the lights only because it has run out of petrol. It responds to a signal, as in a football game which is started and stopped by the referee's whistle. Termination, like activation, involves a combination of inner and outer factors that provide the consummatory conditions it requires. This applies to all purposive behaviour.

The essence of Bowlby's 'attachment behaviour' is that it is seen as part of the total biological system in which the organism is involved, having individual, social and even ecological aspects. It is not the result of 'inner urges', nor is it initially dependent upon physiological needs. It is distinct from feeding and from sexuality, and is of at least equal importance. Its biological significance would seem to derive from the necessity to defend against predators.

The individual is equipped genetically with a balanced repertoire of behavioural potentialities appropriate to each stage of ontogeny. The young require different systems from the adult, but the two are significantly related. Those of mother and child together, for instance, form a stable dyadic system promoting reciprocal attachment.

These views seem far removed from those of psychoanalysis, where Bowlby began. What, one might ask, has become of feeling, of emotion? Bowlby describes subjective experience as a 'phase' of his primary biological events, rather than the central object of analysis. The fact that emotional feeling is associated with instinct cannot be avoided, of course; and acknowledging this in terms of attachment behaviour, he says that when the behaviour is free to reach termination, the 'experience' is an urge to action, while when it is not free there is unease and anxiety, and what to the psychologically-minded could be called an 'unconscious wish'.

During the first 9 months of life, a child's attachment behaviour is not clearly goal-correctable. Terminating conditions are either there, in which case the child is content, or not there, in which case he is distressed; but he is unable to plan his responses. Around 12 months, he begins to 'understand' what conditions terminate the distress, and he is able to plan his behaviour by having 'set goals' towards which his behaviour is guided by feedback control. These plans and goals are specific for particular environments, and are 'set' in conjunction with reciprocal behaviour perceived in the attachment figure. By the end of the first year, he can relate to his 'good' object by appropriate attachment, capable of evoking reciprocal responses, e.g. in mother, with satisfactory consummation. About the same time, his withdrawal from fear-arousing situations – his 'bad' object-relations – has also developed. At first, e.g. around 3 months, the good and bad objects seem separate. Nevertheless in practice it is habitually mother who terminates most of his attachment responses, and proximity to her has become a principal set-goal. This has two important consequences. First, the good and bad partial objects become focused upon a single person, and the child's response becomes an ambivalent attachment as development proceeds. Secondly, as the dyadic system of mother-child develops by reciprocal learning, the child's instinctual attachment becomes quite specific for *his own* mother, not just any kind woman who fulfils his needs. Bowlby makes an important point of this, for which he used the term 'monotropy'. Referring to monotropy, he writes: 'In the human personality, the integrating function of the unique mother-figure is one whose importance cannot be exaggerated.' The development of attachment behaviour in humans is summarised in Volume 1, p 272, of Bowlby's trilogy. The psychiatric problems arising from early maternal deprivation (e.g. delinquency) are attributable to interference with this function. In fact we are dealing here with the development of the ability to relate to another person.

All the attachment responses of childhood have their own beginning, zenith and decline in the course of personal development. They adapt the child to infancy, and fade out when no longer needed. But like old soldiers, they never die. They remain, quite normally, in less prominent states of activity, or of latency; and they can appear again in the adult repertoire, especially at times of stress and danger. This does *not* necessarily indicate pathology, as is implied by the psychoanalytic term 'regression'. Mostly the reappearance is healthy and adaptive. Mourning may be cited as an example of this.

As attachment responses exist, so do the models the child creates in his mind of his attachment figures and their behaviour in relation to himself. These mental models are *working models of what he has experienced*; and they enable him to forecast whether or not his attachment figure is likely to be available and responsive when required. The term 'working models' of objects and self is used because it is more consistent with biology and systems theory than the idea of 'introjected objects and relationships'.

I mentioned mourning as an example of the normal recurrence of early separation responses reappearing in adult life. This touches on one of Bowlby's main contributions to clinical psychiatry, which he set out in his paper 'Processes of Mourning', 1961. Bowlby dealt with this more fully later – in Volume 3 of

'Attachment and Loss'. In our present context this issue need not concern us in detail; but the possibility that attachment can be frustrated raises the very relevant questions of separation, anxiety and anger, which are the subject of Volume 2 of 'Attachment and Loss'.

Again the starting point is empirical observation of children and animals in natural conditions, with experiments and research to investigate fear behaviour: i.e. the methods of ethology. The prototype of anxiety, anger, grief, and defences against these, is seen in the forced *interference with attachment*. For the infant, this means separation from, or absence of, mother. To Bowlby, the basic anxiety is separation-anxiety. The first awareness of separation, as we have seen, comes at the critical period of 28 weeks, when the infant first conceives of himself and mother as separate persons. Ethological data show three elements in the fear response:

(a) Immobility (freezing)
(b) Increased distance from one sort of object (withdrawal)
(c) Decreased distance from another sort of object (attachment)

The involvement of attachment and withdrawal *together* in relation to the same object would generate conflict, should the attachment figure itself elicit fear. The creature then finds itself clinging to a threatening figure. This is the basic example of 'anxious attachment', which will later emerge as a key concept in the thesis.

It is essential to note that each of the stimulus-situations that humans (and animals) are genetically biased to respond to with fear is *a signal of potential danger only*. None need be intrinsically dangerous. For example, the experiences of being in the dark, and hearing a loud noise can induce fear without actually being dangerous. By the same token, each of the stimulus-situations that the child is biased to approach and cling to when he is alarmed is also a *signal*, and does not in itself constitute safety. (This distinction between physical reality and the cues to behaviour reminds us of the analogous distinction between physical need and psychological attachment.) It follows from this that fears of non-dangerous situations are not necessarily 'neurotic'. As he grows up, the child gets used to the signals; and through development and learning, he comes to fit his familiar environment more and more adaptively, whether it be 'good' or 'bad' in the wider context within and beyond the family. Because fears arise from natural cues to which there is instinctive response, and not from real dangers, misattribution and misunderstanding can easily occur. Loud noise is a natural cue – despite reason attributing fear to, for example, lightning rather than thunder. Where two or more stimuli co-exist, one can expect additional fear; yet usually only one of the cues is picked out to signify 'the danger'. Take the example of *being alone, in the dark and hearing a strange noise*. It is nearly always the noise that is picked out, and the other two cues ignored. The noise may then be rationalised into a 'real' danger, such as burglars or ghosts. This mechanism has clear links with so-called 'phobias', where fears appear to be misattributed. We shall examine this later.

Bowlby believes that a vast number of so-called irrational or 'neurotic' fears turn out to be founded on actual fact, if the situation is fully understood. He implies that full investigation of such complaints leave far fewer 'imaginary' fears and dangers (to be accounted for by psychopathology) than most of us realise. Here there is criticism of the psychoanalytic approach. E.g. in the Kleinian system, the child attributes his *own* hostility to the parent, then 'introjects the bad object' (i.e. conceives an inner model of the parent being hostile). Thereafter, the child's anxious relationship is attributed to his own projection of this inner concept on to the real parent, believing it to be objectively true. Not only is this formulation rooted in a non-evolutionary paradigm unrelated to modern biology (Klein's belief in a 'death instinct'), but it directs clinical attention away from real experience, and treats the person as though he were a closed system insulated from his environment. In fact, parents can, and do, evoke real fear, intentionally or unintentionally – but one may not understand the cues.

There are people of all ages who are prone to anxiety, in the sense that they show unusually frequent and urgent attachment behaviour without an apparently adequate cause. They are often pejoratively called immature, neurotic or overdependent, and the cause is sometimes linked with too much indulgence or 'spoiling'. What the actual situation often boils down to is a lack of confidence that the attachment figure will be available when needed: hence the tendency to cling on. Bowlby calls this 'anxious attachment', and it is crucial to his views of psychiatric disturbance. Clinical studies led him to believe that most children's separation fears are reality-bases, either in actual separation experience or in parental threats of abandonment, divorce, suicide, or serious quarrelling.

The child's working models of his attachment figures and of self are built up not just in infancy, but also throughout the years of childhood and adolescence, gradually becoming more fixed with time. The particular forms that a person's working models take are a fair reflection of the types of experience he has had, and may still be having. Certainly his behaviour *may* be explicable only in terms of experience many years ago, but not exclusively so in the psychoanalytic sense.

Bowlby directs us to look particularly at the symptom of *phobia* to clarify his way of thinking. We can distinguish two types of phobia: the monosymptomatic phobias and agoraphobia. The former sufferers tend to be otherwise stable, while the latter are characteristically nervous, anxious, often depressed, and have vaguely-directed fears. The former have been called 'true' phobias, and include those of specific objects, and the latter dubbed 'pseudophobia'. Bowlby's views help to clarify this distinction. In true phobias, what is feared is the *presence* of something frightening. In pseudophobia, what is feared is the *absence or loss* of an attachment figure, or secure base, to which the anxious person would normally retreat. 'School refusal' offers a useful field to study phobic phenomena, and opens the way to understanding some of the interactions between the child and the family system in which he grows up. There are four basic family interaction patterns which Bowlby extracts from the vast literature on the topic of school refusal. These are, in order of frequency:

(1) A pattern where an anxious mother clings to a child, and keeps him at home to comfort herself, without realising her true motive. In her anxious state, she may imagine that she is doing all she can to help him. Such a mother was often herself a victim of insecure attachment in early life, as her history will probably show; and this causes her clinging behaviour, heavily rationalised as care for her poor vulnerable little boy. *The child is presented with a biased image of himself,* as being unfit for the rough world. The true family pattern is camouflaged by an inversion of the parent-child relation. This is a serious anger-provoking situation for the child, while presenting him with no acceptable outlet for his feelings and a denial of their validity.

(2) The child fears disaster to mother and stays at home to prevent it. As opposed to analytical theories of unconscious hostility, Bowlby believes that usually what the child fears arises out of his real experiences. What he fears here is loss of his attachment figure; hence he stays at home, or insists on his attachment figure accompanying him. The fear often arises out of parental quarrels, with mother threatening to walk out, kill herself, become ill, die, or the like. Again, however, it is the child's 'nervousness' that is frequently blamed for the resulting inconvenience.

(3) The child fears disaster to himself, and stays at home to prevent it. Here again actual parental threats are frequently involved, e.g. to send him away for alleged misbehaviour, lock him out of the house, etc.

(4) Mother fears disaster to the child, and keeps him at home. This often results from a belief (whether founded on fact or not) that the child is disabled or 'delicate' – a belief accepted within the family, and perhaps rooted in some tragedy in the family background. In such a case, the child is bearing the brunt of the family's insecurity, and as in the other cases, is being scapegoated.

These family patterns, particularly the first three, are also found in the histories of agoraphobics. For example, an agoraphobic daughter may have a 'dominating and controlling' mother, with whom her relationship is 'close and intense'. The daughter may be described as being 'emotionally immature', the mother as 'overprotective', and their relationship as being one of 'overdependency'. What these emotionally-loaded terms add up to is anxious attachment, with fear of loss in both mother and daughter, with the daughter elected to be the 'patient'. Both are behaving in such a way as to try to ensure that the dreaded separation does not happen. The tone of disparagement in such words as 'immature' and 'overdependent' arises from the old theory of morbid regression, in terms of which anxious attachment is considered infantile, and brought about by treating a child as if he were an infant – i.e. 'spoiling'. This is the exact opposite of what we now see to be the cause. The central position of *fear of loss* in this theory of agoraphobia links it with bereavement and depression. This would account for the panics, irritability and depression so often present. In quite a number of cases bereavement is a precipitating cause.

At this point, one is entitled to ask why, if family interaction is so important in agoraphobia, is it so rarely included as a factor in the initial complaint? Indeed, it is often conspicuously missed out. Of all things, a phobia would seem a specific complaint which the individual person 'has'. First of all, we have already mentioned that when compound situations stimulate fear, involving a number of cues, only one cue tends to be the accepted 'cause'. It will be selected and the other cues suppressed, for some dynamic reason. Here we have an indication of what can occur in families. The family context is suppressed, omitted, or falsified to preserve the family's integrity, and the 'patient' selected as the carrier of the anxiety. This is a very familiar finding in family therapy – the scapegoating of one member. It is made all the easier in the case of a child – who would always prefer to be the 'bad' one himself, and have a 'good' family to depend on, than the other way round. The family is a system; and the more anxious and threatened it feels itself to be, the more it tends in its insecurity to try to maintain itself as a *closed* system. All attempts to explore the pattern, or to interfere or change it are felt as threats, and are resisted. The chosen patient carries all the anxieties disowned by the rest. He is the 'sick' one, while the others are extremely sensitive and defensive. Factors outside the system that can be blamed are eagerly seized upon, such as unsympathetic teachers, bullying boys, dangerous traffic, etc, and are invoked to explain the 'illness'. In this way, phobias are born – to localise and extrude the family problem: and once born, they grow to have a life of their own.

Bowlby proceeds to examine in some detail how the 'patient' himself comes to be unaware, or so confused, regarding the family context of his state. We have seen that a child may idealise the family, often at his own expense. But the situation is usually quite complex. In some more malignant cases, the 'patient' may have been so misled by contradictory information since childhood that he has never known where the truth lay. If the data upon which his working models of attachment figures and self are constructed have been persistently incompatible, he will never know whether his own perception of family reality is true or false. In such an event, there could be several outcomes. He may break with his family – a difficult, and in the circumstances probably irreversible, outcome. Or he may comply with the prevailing family version of reality and disown his own. Both parties will then construe the troubles as due to *his* 'nervous illness', totally unintelligible in the family context. This is the pattern already described in agoraphobia. A third outcome would be an attempt at compromise, with uneasy argument oscillating between the two views: a very unstable state. A fourth possibility would be the desperate attempt to integrate the two views of reality – doomed to failure because they are inherently incompatible. This could lead to cognitive breakdown. Bowlby is among those who believe that some serious mental disorders (psychoses) can be understood as developing from cognitive conflict of this kind in families.

The family context is not only important in this view, it is essential: a *sine qua non* to adequate understanding. And the same or similar processes can be expected in all comparable relationship systems – organisms, families, institutions and societies. Anxiety leads to cutting off from environment, and an attempt to close the system. In so far as this succeeds, the individual, family or institution ceases to be an effective living entity. A child brought up in such a family system will do the same with his own inner distress. He will hold it in, tend to deny its link with the family, or with any real relationships or events, perhaps inventing false ones, or preferring to regard the trouble as his 'illness' – i.e. he creates another closed system. If one can open a way into this, not only will all the fear and anger which is appropriate then appear, but also the appropriate need for secure attachment. One then finds oneself dealing with disturbed feelings, but in a real context, and change has become possible.

Having arrived at dealing with disturbed feelings, it would be helpful to look more closely at Bowlby's views on feelings and emotion. In psychodynamic theories it is usual to regard feelings as the immediate causes of behaviour; and in practice, the language of feeling is used in communicating with patients. In Bowlby's formulation, what have been often rather indiscriminately called 'affects' are regarded as *phases* of an individual's situation-appraisals, either of his own inner state of incipient behaviour (readiness to act), or of the succession of environmental states in which he finds himself. Such appraising processes are an integral part of any control system. In the case of behaviour, they precede and accompany the carrying out of action. Often, but not always, they have the property of being experienced consciously, i.e. 'felt'. As well as intensifying and focusing the appraisal of changing environment and organismal states in the control of behaviour, the appraising processes, in so far as they are felt, provide the individual with a monitoring service regarding his own more or less precise states, urges and interactional situations. At the same time, they provide a valuable communication system with his social companions, because of the accompanying expressions, postures, and incipient movements – a 'body-language' that does not have to be conscious. The affects are not forces, nor things that are felt. What is felt is an aspect or phase of a process; and any way of thinking that tends to reify feeling as if it were an entity in its own right – something that one 'has' – must be regarded as inadmissible. That could lead to a therapist supposing that it is enough to 'let the feelings out', to discharge them as if they were simply a quantity of energy, omitting to determine what situation the patient is appraising. Talking about feelings is pretty useless if it omits the precise situations and relevant actions in which their meaning resides.

Bowlby dismisses the two traditional philosophical schools of thought about mental and physical processes (in this case, feeling and behaviour) as unsatisfactory for his argument – i.e. the Cartesian psycho-physical duality and the epiphenomenalism of the strict behaviourists. Regarding feeling as a natural phase of an appraisal process, he quotes the analogy of redness being a phase of iron when it is heated. He discusses the phases of appraisal processes in cybernetic terms, applying not only to sensory input but also, through feedback, to the changes induced by the behaviour. He concludes that the fact of these processes being experienced as 'felt' seems particularly important if there has to be any *learning*, any reassessment and modification of *standards* of appraisal, or of models of environment and organism, and if there are to be changes in future behaviour. Thus feeling is associated with *focusing of attention where there is need for change.* He reminds us that it is a clinical commonplace that only when a patient becomes emotionally aware of how and what he is feeling can therapeutic change be effected.

Finally, while discussing feeling as a mode of social communication, he stresses the importance of emotion as predictive of behaviour. 'Only if an animal, human or sub-human, is reasonably accurate in assessing the mood of another is he able to participate in social life.' This points to the biological (evolutionary) importance of feeling.

It would be appropriate to end this rough sketch of Bowlby's concepts by referring to the genetic systems model which is his preferred structural model of personality development.

Some biologists have thought, and may still think, that the development of the organism, and through it the entire evolutionary process, is predetermined by the DNA. This implies that biological monster, a closed system: and as Piaget has pointed out, simply cancels the whole idea of evolution. One has to think of a preformed organism impervious to influence from the outside itself. In 1957, C H Waddington, Professor of Animal Genetics in Edinburgh, restored the theory of epigenesis to its rightful place. This states that at conception the organism is not a preformed closed system, but its inborn potentialities emerge in stages as a function of time, as part of the wider system that includes its environment. Waddington was thorough-going, and established the role of the environment in 'setting problems' to which genotypical variations are a response. This gives evolution the dialectical character without which it would be an eternally predestined plan strewn with meaningless accidents. Waddington has shown that environment and gene interact in the formation of the phenotype – which is the reaction of the gene complex to environmental influence. He views the relationship between organism and environment as a cybernetic loop, such that the organism selects its environment while being conditioned by it – a process that has some relevance to our topic.

The gene complex exerts control over the interactional processes that determine an organism's development. In particular, there is control over the extent to which each developmental feature is 'environmentally stable' or 'environmentally labile'. Bias towards the stable end would ensure persistent development in the face of a great deal of environmental change, at the price of total inability to tolerate change beyond a certain limit. At the labile end (of high sensitively) there is great adaptability, with the organism varying its developmental tendencies to suit changes in the prevailing environment; but here there is a risk of seriously maladaptive forms arising to some (or all) environments. Because of this risk, epigenetic sensitivity has come to be controlled, or 'buffered', by physiological and behavioural processes that have evolved to modify the impact of environment on species; and acting in concert, these processes tend to keep an individual as nearly as possible on whatever developmental pathway he is already on, despite most environmental fluctuations. Waddington called this method of autoregulation 'homeorhesis', and it brings us back to personality development, because Bowlby sees it as applying to the whole process of an individual's development, from the zygote in the uterine wall to the child within the family, to personality as well as to physical structure. Most psychodynamic models of personality development have taken what one might call the 'single-track railway' form, with its series of stages on the single way to maturity. Stoppage of the train, or 'fixation' of part of it at stations on the way, could occur. Then, for development to proceed, a return to this point, or 'regression', would have to happen later to re-integrate the train. An alternative to this limited notion is the model based on Waddington's idea of a whole system of possible alternative tracks, beginning close together, then branching and diverging as time goes on, yet by the 'points' and 'signals' systems of homeorhesis, progress is effectively controlled according to conditions obtaining, so that the trains can *change routes* if obstructed, yet tend to be kept moving as close to their intended route as possible. This avoids the notion of 'regression' as being necessary for overcoming obstacles to development. So one may envisage the fundamental characteristics of personality development as involving a set of possible alternative pathways on the way to maturity. Which ones are chosen depends upon a number of variables no doubt; but of these, the influences of the family stand out because of their powerful and far-reaching effect. Starting during the first months in his relationship with mother, and extending through childhood and adolescence within the family system, the child builds up and modifies models in himself of how the people he needs are likely to behave towards him in a variety of possible situations; and this intimately affects the way he himself behaves. And on these models are based all his expectation, and therefore all his plans, for the rest of his life. In so far as homeorhetic pressures operate, they come from outside and inside, and tend to maintain the status quo of developmental direction. As a consequence, it may be difficult or impossible to treat a developing child outside the family context. The older he grows, the more resistant his developmental processes become to the influences of environmental change, and the less modifiable his internal working models; so that comparatively little modification takes place after adolescence. As for the individual's own homeorhetic resistance to developmental change, we recognise it in the phenomena known to psychiatrists as the 'mechanisms of defence'. Unlike the older theory of 'regression', this model denies that adult neurotic patterns are resurgences of reactions that were normal in childhood, or that the behaviour indicates a return to immaturity. As will be clear from this theoretical model, Bowlby insists that psychodynamic theory should conform to the principles of developmental biology and evolution, and that one should be wary of using the medical conceptions of pathology to account for variations in behaviour.

In his chapter on family influences upon child disturbances in Emanuel Miller's book on Child Psychiatry, Ackerman expresses some very relevant views. He traces the concepts of family interaction from older atomistic ideas to modern holistic ones. He then undertakes a critique of the psychoanalytic attitude, which he sees as preoccupied with parts rather than with the whole. He then asks: 'How far does the child's personality unfold autonomously from within, and how far is its development influenced from without? This is the riddle of the inner and outer faces of personality: the mystery of the relations of subject and object, the I and me.' At once we recognise the familiar problems of epigenesis we have just been looking at in general biological terms. Here they are appearing at the very root of personality development. Referring to what he calls 'the inner and outer faces of personality', Ackerman says that in psychoanalytical theory one cannot be clear how far they are joined and how far they are separate. In this he seems to me to echo some of Bowlby's misgivings. Psychoanalysis reveals how the child's image of his family may involve falsification – see Melanie Klein – but not how a child assimilates his correctly perceived experience of the realities of family interaction. Bowlby upholds the importance of the *actual* environment as a *cause*, against the current of psychoanalytic tradition; and he believes in the essential reciprocity of responses between subject and object, regarding them as inseparable in the growth of object relations and the development of personality.

List of researchers:

Balint, Alice
Balint, Michael
Erikson, Erik
Fairbairn, Ronald
Ferenczi, Sandor
Freud, Sigmund
Hartmann, Heinz

Hermann, Nunberg
Hinde, Robert
Klein, Melanie
Lorenz, Konrad
Piaget, Jean
Robertson, James and Joyce
Schaffer, H Rudolph
Spitz, Rene
Sullivan, Harry Stack
Waddington, C H (Professor of Animal Genetics, Edinburgh)
Winnicott, D W

Bowlby, J Int J Psychoanalysis, 39, 1958 'The Nature of the Child's Tie to Mother.'
Bowlby J 'Attachment and Loss' volume 1 and 'The Child's Tie to Mother.'
Bowlby J 'Processes of Mourning' (paper) 1961, and in volume 3 of 'Attachment and Loss'.
Miller, Emanuel 'Foundations of Child Psychiatry' (also chapter by Nathan Ackerman)
Shaffer H R 'Some issues for Research in the Study of Attachment Behaviour', p179 of 'Determinants of Infant Behaviour', Ed Foss.

Piagetian Theory and Psychodynamics

"If the sciences of nature explain the human species, humans in turn explain the sciences of nature."
(Piaget)

As is characteristic of most scientific endeavour, it seems reasonable for us to try to create a more unified theory than we already have of mental development and mental functioning, particularly one which would bring the cognitive and the psychodynamic systems together as part of a general biological principle. Some separate attempts have already been made to reach a biological basis. For example, the psychoanalyst John Bowlby has gone far to integrate psychodynamics with biology by adopting ethological methods, and by incorporating the principle of cybernetics and the epigenetic ideas of C H Waddington. In parallel with this, Jean Piaget has done likewise with the cognitive mental function (and has acknowledged the same sources). Yet in spite of these tendencies one cannot help feeling uneasy that psychodynamic theory takes so little account of cognitive factors, while cognitively-based systems such as Piaget's take so little notice of psychodynamics. It ought surely to be possible to bring both of them together under the same biological umbrella.

Inhelder described Piaget as 'a zoologist by training, an epistemologist by vocation and a logician by method' and this triple orientation is undoubtedly reflected throughout his work. He has been concerned primarily with the nature of knowledge and its biological significance, so he draws attention to the close connection between vital (biological) mechanisms and cognitive ones. In a major work 'Biology and Knowledge' he writes: 'All knowledge, in fact, of whatever nature it may be, raises the

27

problem of the relations between subject and object; and this problem can lead to many solutions according to whether one attributes such knowledge to the subject alone, to an action by the object, or to the interactions of both. Now, since the subject is one aspect of the organism, and the object a sector, as it were, of the environment, the problem of knowledge seen from this point of view corresponds to the problem of the relations between the organism and the environment – undeniably the most general question in the whole of biology. Equally undeniable is the way this question keeps cropping up; and every time it arises there arise with it a series of possible solutions, each as different from the other as are the epistemological or the psychogenetic ones.' So Piaget describes cognitive function ('knowledge') as an aspect of the major biological problem of relation between organism and environment; and of course we acknowledge that the psychodynamic aspect of life is another. We then have the biological question of organism and environment embracing the epistemological question of subject knowing about object (Piaget's basic concern) and also the psychodynamic question of ego relation to object, which is most easily construed, in this biological context, in terms of Bowlby's ethological formulation and Fairbairn's object-relations theory. It is the relation of Piaget's psychology to Fairbairn's that has particularly interested me, and I propose here to deal with some aspects of the possible unification of these two views.

What first appealed to me on approaching Piaget was his ethologically based starting point; and in the realm of theory, his taking the 'action schema' as the basic atom from which mental life is built up. We can consider the subject-object relation in terms of three aspects of the subject: (1) the biological 'organism', (2) the cognitive 'mind', and (3) the psychodynamic 'ego'. In all these aspects the relation is founded on a dynamic structure which is active, and dynamically orientated from the start. For Piaget, the first representation of the outer world of objects is of the *response* of the organism in interaction with these objects. Here is no 'pure' observation, no mere acceptance nor passive reflection of the world. The organism that adapts, the mind that knows and (if I might here add to Piaget's system) the ego that relates, represent an active agent from the beginning *creatively involved* with the reality it adapts to, and knows, and seeks in relationship. Piaget's views therefore differ from those earlier ones which considered the primary mental awareness to be simply perception of the object in an initially uninvolved and passive way, implying an essential separateness between ego and object (cf. William James's 'empirical observing self'). Piaget's theory states that the actual awareness of an object *qua* object *develops out of action schemata, quite late*, by a process of differentiation. This happens at about 7 months of age, which accords with the separation-anxiety period of Spitz and Bowlby.

In considering this intimate interacting quality of the first awareness of reality at the very inception of mind, one is really assuming some sort of *a priori* congruence between subject and object. An organism does not interact with just any object. It interacts with those objects which are already there in relation to it when it comes into being. Normally a creature is born into the environment within which its genetic structure has already evolved. The human infant (and its analogue, the primitive ego) comes into being within an environment of evolutionary adaptedness – what Hartmann called its 'average expectable environment'. And because of the already existing mutual suitedness, the new organism interacts with an environment, and with specific objects therein, to which it is designed to adapt. The potential sensorimotor responses, the 'instinctual' behaviour, object-seeking and general adaptations function appropriately from the start, because of the genetic evolutionary process in which they are embedded. In a sense, the potential *relation* between organism and environment, between ego and object, is there before they arise as separate constructs at all. Piaget quotes a colleague as once saying 'In the beginning was the Response!' Thereafter the action schemata ensure a relationship that becomes more and more closely adapted, more epistemologically meaningful and more psychodynamically necessary.

These three levels, the biological, the cognitive and the psychodynamic, correspond to the aspects of the living subject already referred to. Piaget has little to say about the last of these. He does not use the ego-relationship terminology that I have introduced, although so far it seems to fit his trend of thought. He talks rather about organismal need in the sense of 'need to function'. He writes: 'The psychological need for an object is the result of contact with that object, and the need persists until the behaviour has been adapted to the novelty.' Again: 'The basic fact is not need as such, but rather the act of assimilation which embodies functional need, repetition and coordination between subject and object in the one whole.' Notice that despite his chosen cognitive framework, Piaget is always thinking in dynamic, relational terms. Biologically, the force motivating behaviour lies in the innate tendency to respond functionally, inherent in inherited dynamic structures that have arisen to maintain life within its accustomed environment. A living thing draws on its environment to preserve and develop itself in a state of structural separateness from that environment through a specific dependency upon it. When initial primitive sensorimotor reflexes occur, the organism (e.g. human infant) strives to repeat them. A 'need to function' has been released. The infant who has had a grasp- or sucking-reflex deliberately or accidentally stimulated, strives to relate in this way again, grasping or sucking whatever new objects present themselves. This primitive awareness of reality *by acting upon it* is the atomic basis from which mind is built up, and Piaget called it the 'action schema'. By repetition, the child continues to assimilate new objects into his existing action schemata, extending his range of experience by applying his simple methods of responding. Frequently, however, this does not work; so a second function of the action schema comes into play. Accidentally or deliberately he finds that some modification of the schema makes his goal more readily achievable. This constitutes *accommodation*.

By assimilation the child seeks to make reality suit his own functioning; by accommodation he adapts his functioning to suit reality. In this way the action schemata become more flexible and adaptive, ensuring a progression of development.

Piaget describes the child's development as a succession of interconnected stages, each stage transcending the preceding one, yet still incorporating its potentialities. No stage can be attained without passing through its predecessors. Following Waddington, he proposes that this is a fundamental biological principle, and that in biological epigenesis this process of development is set by the genome. The effect of the environment upon the developing organism is so regulated by this genetic influence that each stage has its own environmental sensitivity, so to speak. That is, the environment can only influence development to the degree allowed for at each particular stage. At other stages that particular influence would have no significant effect. E.g. a child can learn to count when he is at a certain epigenetic stage; before that, he would be unreceptive to the concept. The evolving phenotype is not impervious to environmental influences, but the effect is regulated stage by stage. In the broad evolutionary sense, as Waddington put it, the environment 'sets problems to which genotypical variations are a response'. Environment and genome interact in the formation of the phenotype in this controlled way – a cybernetic loop, as it were. This implies a dialectical process, a two-way influence, in which the organism comes to select its environment as well as being influenced by it. There is a clear structural similarity here to Piaget's ideas of assimilation and accommodation. The control exercised by the gene complex determines in particular the extent to which each developmental feature is 'environmentally stable' or 'environmentally labile'. Bias towards the stable end ensures persistent development despite great environmental change, at the price of total inability to tolerate change beyond a certain limit. At the labile end (high sensitivity), there is great adaptability to environmental changes, but with the risk of serious distortion and of maladaptive forms arising in some environments. Because of these risks, buffering systems have evolved to stabilise the developmental process as it interacts with the environment. Acting in concert, these physiological and behavioural processes tend to keep the individual on whatever developmental pathway he is already on (or as nearly as possible) despite environmental fluctuations. Waddington called this mode of autoregulation 'homeorhesis'.

These ideas were adopted by Piaget in his biological stance. The earliest stage he called the 'sensorimotor phase' of mental development, and he divided this into six sub-stages that characterise the first 18 months of life. During this time the schemata become more autonomous as mental patterns, more flexible and 'mobile' – i.e. capable of being applied generally to situations with which they had not been originally involved. Here we have the beginning of true *mental* functioning. 'Action' can be seen as something the child can not only do, but can *will* to do, rather than a mere automatic response. The child's repertoire of schemata now begins to constitute what we may call an 'ego'. By about seven to eight months, a conscious distinction can be made between the acting self and the object that was not possible before. The schemata have become so numerous, mobile and varied that it is possible to define the object as an invariant. Hence the environment is conserved. At the same time the schemata have become so generally applicable that they define a willing and acting self. This marks the beginning of awareness of the permanent externality of the objective world. And as the object is stripped of its subjective action content, and is seen to be unchangingly 'out there', so the action is liberated from its tie to specific objects and is conceived of as 'this is me'. This is the so-called period of separation-anxiety already referred to. The world is now seen to be separate from the self, with a will of its own. From this point exploratory behaviour becomes possible and finally real inventiveness, not just trial and error. So we have the establishment of a true inner mental world. Action can be taken mentally, or considered and rehearsed, without having to use objects physically. Action by the end of this phase can be internalised as mental activity; and the world has its inner counterpart in 'thought schemata' that have evolved by integration and coordination of the primitive action phases. Assimilation and accommodation become differentiated from each other. Accommodation becomes an end in itself, leading to novel experiences. Experiences can be assimilated into thought schemata, so that mental attitudes grow to be ever more realistically orientated. This means that behaviour can become increasingly appropriate and adaptive before it is put into effect at all, and means of accommodation can be considered which are no longer inevitably limited to what is being immediately acted upon.

Even by the end of the sensorimotor period, however, the capacity to conserve reality internally in thought schemata is limited to immediate surroundings only, and is relatively short-lived unless contact with objects is repeatedly re-established to provide 'aliment' to keep the schemata going. I understand by Piaget's word 'aliment' the satisfaction of the need to function – what it is that makes assimilation 'desirable': the consummatory completion of an activated schema. Theoretically one might perceive here the primitive beginnings of affectivity. Piaget's sensorimotor postulate considers affective and intellectual development as two aspects of the same process. His view was that intelligence has three aspects – cognition, perception and affectivity. He wrote: 'The development of intelligence is a unitary process pertaining to all aspects of mental development, including sensorimotor intelligence, perception, cognition and affectivity. All of mental development starts with motor activity, all motor activity is intentional and object-directed, and the end result of all motor activity is the establishment of stable mental processes – the schemata – which are the basis of intelligent thought.'

Following the sensorimotor phase of the first 18 months of life, Piaget describes another three stages that need not detain us long. With the development of true representational schemata

33

there open out the preconceptual and the intuitive sub-stages (seen in imitation, play, games with rules) leading to the beginning of conceptual thinking. There follows the period of 'concrete operations', where logical thinking is possible, but still requires a concrete basis, and finally we have the stage of 'formal operations' where logico-mathematical thinking can occur, and the mind is finally freed from its original action-based tie to the concrete object.

This is a very sketchy summary of the considerable richness of Piaget's developmental psychology, emphasising the sensorimotor period because that would seem to have the most relevance in a psychodynamic context. In the decade 1956-66, E J Anthony argued that psychiatry generally had a lot to gain from a study of Piaget, and that clinical work, especially with children, could benefit from his ideas, e.g. of animism, egocentrism and object permanence. He believed that clinical evidence supported many of Piaget's theories. However, the main study to date that set out to link Piagetian theory with psychodynamics was Peter Wolff's book 'The Developmental Psychologies of Jean Piaget and Psychoanalysis', written in 1960. He sets Piaget's ideas out side-by-side with 'classical' psychoanalysis (libido theory, etc) and attempts a synthesis – finding the way smoothed by Erikson's social emphasis and Hartmann's ego psychology.

It had seemed to me that the object-relations theory of Fairbairn and the ethological approach of Bowlby might lead to a more fruitful unification of Piagetian and psychodynamic theory. Thinking of the difference between the affects and satisfactions of interest and curiosity associated with action schemata and the power and persistence of those associated with primary human object-attachment, I wondered if 'interpersonal schemata' did not perhaps exist in a class of their own. I then discovered that this had been thought of already, and a paper had been written in 1975 by Robert W Goldberg on this very topic – 'Piagetian Theory and the Helping Professions': Proceedings of an Interdisciplinary Seminar, University of South California, 1975. So what follows owes much to his work.

It is surely not necessary here to review Fairbairn's theories in detail. Let us just mention that he proposed *relationship* rather than the press of Freudian 'instincts' as the key factor in development. There is an innate impulsion towards relationship with certain objects in the environment. Although lacking any experience of external reality as such to begin with, the child is reality-orientated from the outset. What is instinctively sought is interaction with a person, not pleasurable discharge of libido. When a satisfactory relationship favouring equilibrium and smooth development is frustrated, the child may try to overcome the obstacle (Piaget – 'accommodation of schemata'). But failing this, he gives up on reality and takes the frustrating problem into his mind, and tries to deal with it there, because day-to-day life has to go on round him regardless, and the world does not stop until he gets things straightened out. This internalisation Fairbairn called (after Klein) 'introjection of the bad object' in its relation to a frustrated-needy part of the ego unable to detach from it. The introject is a dynamic structure of ego-acting-on-object (more accurately part-ego acting on part-object) with the goal of making that 'bad' part of reality assimilable (to use Piaget's phrase). If object relationships are benign and satisfying on the whole, then fuller development and psychic differentiation between a relatively unitary ego and the external object will continue. Fairbairn does not say much about this aspect of emotional life – the world of the 'central ego'. The internalised schemata described by Piaget are not considered. He maintains that so long as the child is satisfied and his central ego system remains open to interaction with an environment of predominantly 'good' objects, he gets on with his life and his development without the internalising process (here called introjection) being necessary. It is only if maternal care, for example, is not good enough, or too exciting-frustrating, or too rejecting, that the child cannot cope with his objects in real life, and he has to take the whole process of the blocked relationship into his mind and try to deal with it there. So introjection of the bad object occurs. On a psychological level, this is an attempt to cope magically (regressively) by making the bad good when coping realistically has failed. But biologically there is an underlying adaptive significance which Piaget would perhaps recognise, namely an attempt to find new ways of coping with an obstacle to development, even although the mental means is not yet to hand. The means becomes available at a later epigenetic stage, with the development of 'mobile' action schemata and the ability to represent reality mentally, to explore and try out new behaviours (at around 12 to 16 months of age – the 5th stage of sensorimotor development).

In Piaget, the analogue of 'bad relation' is an interactional situation where assimilation to an existing motor schema is not possible, because the situation is too remote from previous experience for adaptation to occur at the particular epigenetic level at the time. The important internalisation for Piaget is that of 'good' (assimilable) objects, while for Fairbairn the opposite applies, as we have seen. As a doctor he has been most concerned with pathology.

These are important differences of emphasis; but let us now look at some of the aspects the two views have in common.

First observation: *The elements of the psyche are dynamic structures.*

Both theories postulate basic mental structures that involve dynamic interaction between subject and object. Although in each theory the nature of the structures, and their significance for the whole, change epigenetically during development, from the outset the structures possess the capacity to function on their own. Although Piaget said little about the affective aspect of schemata, Wolff in his comparison with psychoanalysis elaborated the notion of 'affective schemata' to cover sensorimotor action systems where action is blocked, and there are strong 'affect discharges'. As with action, the affect is assimilated into an innate schema, and the child may respond by screaming with rage, for example.

Presumably the affect schemata develop like the others, and most become integrated with the whole system. Moreover these mental developments are occurring as part of an essential interpersonal context as far as affect is concerned, because emotional expression is a non-verbal signal system of great social importance. The human beings around the child, such as mother, to whom he has always been in relation, act as autonomous causal agents, and also respond selectively to the child's affective expression of need, hunger, anger, etc, as well as pleasure, curiosity, interest and cleverness. Similarly for Fairbairn, Winnicott and Bowlby, affective expression is thought of in this way, and is inherent in the ego structures.

So we might hypothesise that at birth infants possess a number of inherited functional structures, which may be activated in an average expectable environment (Hartmann) and 'released' by the human and non-human objects therein. Some of the resulting behaviour is associated with 'drive affect' (Wolff) – strong and persistent; other behaviour with milder 'interest' affects (Piaget).

Second observation: *There exists a range of possible ways of experiencing relationships.*

Fairbairn's emphasis is on the importance of 'bad' relationships – too 'exciting' or too frustrating. Piaget's emphasis is on interactions that are satisfying, 'interesting' or at least tolerable.

So we might hypothesise that there is a *continuum* of experience from the highly exciting at one end through a satisfying zone to the highly frustrating at the other: the mid-section of experience being tolerable.

Third observation: *There exists some process of 'internalisation' of reality.*

This applies to both Piaget's assimilation and Fairbairn's introjection. Some sort of mental representation of the object, however primitive, is in the process of formation, and may be stabilised by repeated experience. For Fairbairn there need be no internalisation unless relationship is unsatisfactory; for Piaget, the ground relationship is at least tolerable and assimilation satisfying. Each emphasises opposite conditions. Moreover their targets differ: Fairbairn the interpersonal world, Piaget the impersonal.

Here we might hypothesise that throughout the range of experiences of relationship noted above, the internalisation that occurs is a basically normal process, not necessarily a pathological one. There is a mental registration of experiences with human objects (cf Bowlby's 'working models') which contributes to the formation and growth of the schemata – the dynamic structures – whether the relationship is satisfying or not, no matter how rudimentary the ego is, or how primitive its ability to deal with the experiences.

Fourth observation: *There are internal structural linkages, formed between aspects of the ego and its representation of the human object.*

This is made quite explicit in object-relations theory, in Fairbairn's postulation of 'partial egos'. Here the unassimilable fragments of unsatisfied ego and bad object combined become split off from mainstream development of self-in-reality, and form closed systems that can no longer develop or be changed. Piaget has not, so far as I know, dealt with personal interaction as a specific dynamic in the formation of schemata, although he does seem to view the development of relationships with people as parallel to, and integrated with, cognitive development. One such reference concerns his notion of 'decentring'. By this he means the child ceasing to relate everything to himself, his own state and his own actions. He says that when cognitive decentring occurs, affective decentring comes with it. The child can then know that other people can have their own feelings. At this stage he can grasp external reality more as a whole, rather than as consisting only of the parts he perceives while inferring the rest on the basis of pre-existing schemata.

We are now perhaps in a position to make another hypothesis: An important type of structure is directly formed by the interaction of the infant's schemata with the reaction of others to him. The linked cognitive and affective experiences of the child-and-others relationship appears to be very powerful in our species, and in Piaget's terminology provides important 'interpersonal aliment' for the formation of *interpersonal schemata* (Goldberg). In the evolution of these, some aspect of the object's emotional attitude to the child is reacted to, and mentally registered in a manner limited by the level of epigenetic development – cognitive and affective. In this type of schema, the emotional-behavioural presence of the object is the Gestalt 'focus' of the interaction as is the case in Fairbairn's theory, rather than the background to it as it usually is with Piaget. The 'interpersonal schemata' which Goldberg proposes (and I second him) are continuous structures, having their inherited precursors, their elementary forms in the paranatal period, subsequently integrating, differentiating and modifying through experience like the cognitive schemata. For the interpersonal schemata, perhaps the ultimate phase of 'formal operations' represents the ability to see other people wholly without preconceptions, personal bias or projection, and to allow them freedom to be themselves.

However, to return to the prototype relation of child to mother, we can now usefully compare Piaget's and Fairbairn's views. Let us take the behaviour of sucking. For Piaget, *the child ready to suck meets a nipple.* As he acts on it, there is progressively greater efficiency and improved bodily conformity of both child and mother. Moreover, the release of this behaviour is affectively satisfying. For Piaget, much of this satisfaction is because the child has succeeded in acting adaptively in relation to a cooperating other. Now consider the situation for Fairbairn. *The child does not have the nipple, but needs it.* He is excited and frustrated until he gets it. If he does not get it, he becomes distressed and adopts the defence mechanism of introjection. Unlike Piaget, Fairbairn's interest centres on the *failure* to consummate the interpersonal act when considering its developmental significance. The failure to act adaptively leads to aspects of the 'bad' object-relationship being split off, and these persist unmodified 'in the unconscious', as psychoanalysts say. This state of affairs is also familiar to Piaget, whose schemata, without aliment (without successful exercise), cannot be sustained or built upon, but remain unchanged.

To the extent that the infant cannot perform the actions required by the nature of interpersonal schemata (i.e. there is an exciting-but-frustrating object), these schemata will remain in their rudimentary state and will not be able to develop. Moreover, since the infant cannot act on interpersonal reality, there is a failure of differentiation of self and object. For Piaget this means the failure of assimilation and accommodation to separate, and for Fairbairn, failure to leave the position of primary identification.

Thus it is concluded that interpersonal schemata consisting of intolerable (impossible) ego-object actions and affects are not subject to further normal development. Key experiences (e.g. a good enough maternal response) have not occurred at critical periods, so that the rudimentary schemata have remained in an 'open' state (i.e. without aliment: without anything to act on). They are 'unterminated', in the language of attachment theory. In this state they cannot be integrated with other structures operative at that particular developmental stage; but they continue unterminated, to function in their primitive rudimentary way – continually unsuccessfully – and because of this they can, and do, colour later relationships. For example, a psychiatric patient may attempt to relate emotionally to others as if they represented the nipple he never had, but still seeks. However, trying to provide compensatory experiences in later life may be of no help, because they are being applied out of epigenetic context – i.e. not at the developmental stage where they were needed. However, to the extent that other persons (his objects) do permit the infant to perform consummatory actions according to the nature of his interpersonal schemata, these schemata will stabilise, differentiate more clearly, develop further and integrate with other appropriate schemata. This is in line with Piaget's view of how the child builds up notions of 'realistic' objects – the meaning of 'realistic' being determined by the phase of cognitive development he is at, e.g. sensorimotor, concrete operations, etc. Bowlby's attachment theory comes to conclusions almost identical to this.

So it would seem that the general rules provided by Piaget for the differentiation and integration of schemata might be extended beyond the cognitive into the interpersonal psychodynamic realm. For instance, Melanie Klein believes that at about 6 months the child begins to realise that the 'good' and 'bad' mothers, as experienced, are really the same person. This can be taken as the integration of initially separate rudimentary interpersonal schemata, clustered about satisfying and frustrating experiences. In similar fashion, interpersonal schemata might differentiate, so that the infant begins to react differently to separate people originally treated as if they were the same object, but now responded to individually as mother, father, strangers, etc.

It is also to be noted that interpersonal schemata developing within object-relationships that are relatively tolerable do so diachronically: that is, they evolve through time, and allowing for some differentiation and integration, they retain a general historical and functional continuity. The specific human objects that aliment them would remain the same, although the objects' behaviour would certainly change both as they develop and as the child himself changes. With these changes pressing upon the schemata, new aspects are assimilated; and there is also a groping for new ways of relating to objects, i.e. fresh accommodation. In Piaget's terms, the result is a relative equilibrium. However, we remember that when relationships produce too much anxiety, interpersonal schemata remain open and interminable, with resulting disequilibrium of the personality system, and the clinician observes 'regressive', 'defensive' or other so-called pathological ways of relating to others that go on and on.

We have previously referred to the developmental state where self and object are first perceived to be separate entities; and we saw in this separation a new flexibility, the possibility of exploratory behaviour and freedom from total external control. It is this nuclear event that makes psychotherapy possible. When the 'blocks' we have been describing appear at later stages and cannot then be corrected by simple reparatory means, correction can be effected if the mind can be induced to access once more the former experiential states in which these blocks arose. Even although the original blocking events are no longer present, this access can be achieved by therapeutic means, by bringing about the mental state of regression, in which the former affects are re-experienced. A crucial aspect of regression is the loss of personal autonomy, as Piaget has pointed out. Here we think of autonomy as freedom from the 'instinctual drives' of classical Freudianism. From the regressed position, the person can no longer act realistically in the present mature situation from which he has regressed. He has left the adaptive means behind in moving to the lower epigenetic level in which he is bound to the object. This loss of autonomy entails seeing present-day relationships as if they were once again of the old binding, controlling type of the earlier level. We have here arrived at the crucial psychodynamic phenomenon of 'transference', deduced from Piagetian theory. Intervention at this crucial point can be effective because it is then epigenetically appropriate, and the changes can then allow assimilation to occur as treatment removes the blocks.

Psychodynamics had its origin in the study of neurosis and frustrated developmental processes. Hence the theoretical formulations of the therapists – Freud, Klein and Fairbairn, for example – are founded on studies of disturbed conditions. Piaget had no such psychiatric bias, and studied normal children, particularly his own. We have made an attempt here to narrow the gap between medically-based theories and those like Piaget's that arise from observing ordinary behaviour. We may join Goldberg in hoping that these and similar attempts might help towards a theory that does not see object-relationships as *essentially* determined by conflicts of the past, but also as creative adaptations of a developing individual within a realistic interpersonal world.

Of course, this does not mean that the most valuable insights of psychodynamic theory and therapeutic practice have to be sacrificed on the altar of strict biological realism. In evolving his attachment theory, Bowlby has moved far in that direction from his psychodynamic beginnings. Despite the real value of his approach (which has come closer than most to Piaget) he has, in my view, left too much of the psychodynamic *mind* out of the picture. The awareness of a personal Self is at least as real as the reductively-derived concepts of scientific biology, and is implicit in everything we have discussed about mind. We cannot neglect the *subject* of knowing and feeling and acting. It is the Self, the psychodynamic ego, that is chiefly concerned in cognition and epistemology. Without it they would be nothing.

List of researchers:

Anthony, E J
Bowlby, John
Erikson, Erik
Fairbairn, Ronald
Goldberg, Robert W
Hartmann, Heinz
James, William
Klein, Melanie
Spitz, Rene
Waddington, C H
Winnicott, D W

B Inhelder, B (1967) Biology and Knowledge.
Wolff, Peter (1960) The Developmental Psychologies of Jean Piaget and Psychoanalysis.

Dyadic Interaction in Marital Conflict

Psychodynamic processes are concerned with *personal interaction*, and are all derived from the relationships between a person and the significant others to whom he has been, and is, attached. Thus, intrapsychic emotional events such as conflict within the self arise from former eventful interpersonal relationships that have left traces. Hence psychotherapy has to be about what goes on between people – and this includes the client and his or her therapist. It has little or nothing to do with an 'objective' doctor tinkering with a faulty psychic machine, as it were. To exemplify this point, I want to introduce some of the ideas of H V Dicks on the theory of marital interaction, and discuss some of these. To limit a wide field, I shall pick out the topic of conflict in marriage, how it arises, and what are the specifically marital processes we find at work in the psychotherapy of couples.

Dicks and his colleagues worked in marital therapy at the Tavistock Clinic for some 16 years and studied 2000 cases, setting down their ideas in his book 'Marital Tensions', which represents pioneer work in this field. His objective was to view the marriage itself as the core of the problem rather than to treat the two individuals separately. The marriage then emerges as a dyadic entity with a pathology of its own, in which the problems of the individuals are inextricably involved.

He first makes the point that marriage is a social institution *sui generis* – an expression of the prevailing culture's attitude to relational needs between the sexes and of children. At the same time it is also a system of very personal inter-relation – one of the most personal we know – between two people, stable to the degree that it can transform the 1+1 pair into an integrated dyad, amounting to a 'dyadic personality', in which a preponderance of the needs of each partner is satisfied (which incidentally does not imply freedom from conflict, or even happiness).

Going on to examine this dyadic structure, three major sub-systems appear to be involved, and these are investigated in detail:

Sub-systems:
1. Social norms
2. Individual values
3. Unconscious needs

Sub-system 1 is the 'public' system of socio-cultural values and norms, expressing traditional attitudes of social homogeneity. Problems can arise here with culturally exogamous marriages that depart from such norms as race, religion, class, philosophy, etc.

Sub-system 2 is that of individual personal norms: conscious values and expectations, derived from upbringing and social learning in the personal environment. Conflict can arise on this level from divergencies of habits, tastes, etc. and from differences of opinion or interests; but these are unlikely to be serious unless the next sub-system is involved.

Sub-system 3 is the area of unacknowledged unconscious object-relational needs: the products of repressed, unresolved interpersonal conflicts during early development.

To make this clear, let us look for a moment at the psychological processes involved. Object-relational interaction during early development moves from the primary phases of dependence on mother to more differentiated transactions. According to the intensity of conflict during any such phase, the pathways of dynamic flow between self and object are either more or less open along the appropriate developmental line, or are deflected by the (unresolved) conflict into alternative channels whose direction deviates significantly from that line. These constitute the so-called 'split-off' ego-object relations within the self, as described by Fairbairn. These elements remain in their undeveloped state because of their isolation in the unconscious; but primitive regressive interaction within the marital dyad can access them, whereupon they give rise to ambivalent bonding between the partners, and a deeply collusive mutual dependency arises, with all the features and psychodynamic mechanisms familiar in psychotherapy. In health, interaction at this level can provide the opportunity for growth through working through the emerging problems; but if disturbance is severe, quite florid psychiatric disorder can arise at this level, yet can be contained there – i.e. not appearing outside the marriage relationship. It is the state of this sub-system that forms the deep core of marital life, and determines the long-term stability of the dyad both in health and disorder.

These three sub-systems afford us a guide to the general areas in which marital conflict can arise and grow, viz.:

Social setting:
(a) Family structure in a changing environment.
(b) The changing mutual status of men and women.
(c) Culture distance in mate selection:
    e.g. multiracial problems.

Individual setting:
This includes the psychopersonal values: e.g. ego-strength and secure identity that have resulted from individual personal development.

Unconscious needs:
I.e. the area of marital psychopathology, as we might call it, which includes those specifically marital defensive systems employed by the dyad to deal with deep personal conflict.

Let us consider these in a little more detail.

Social setting

(a) Family structure.
Here we note that vastly powerful forces of social change impinge upon the family. At the same time, it is the chief attitude-forming centre of the community, feeding back and forth the results of personal interaction between individuals and the larger society. The social stresses have increased enormously with the disruption of the centuries-old traditional family structure since the Industrial Revolution. Because of culture-lag, we are still suffering from the effects of this drastic change. The traditional extended family was highly structured, and supported by universal, rigid social laws believed to be divinely ordained. It was oppressive, reactionary and static; but also emotionally secure because there was no choice, so reducing the possibility of conflict. Within their prescribed limits, everyone was emotionally secure.

The modern urban family stands in the greatest possible contrast to this. With its few children and relative isolation in an impersonal community, it is a 'vestigial shrunken successor' (Dicks) of the large, close traditional group, with none of its monolithic security. In the narrow confines of this tiny group, all the expectations and needs that used to be met by the traditional family have somehow to be expressed, and somehow met. This implies that the mate is *unconsciously expected* to contain all the role potentials of a large ideal group, and the couple have to be almost literally 'all in all' to each other. Add to this the insecurity and monotony of modern industrial life, and the rat-race, and one can see how so many couples develop a tremendous unsatisfied dependence upon each other, and how children can become the scapegoats for their parents' overflowing unfulfilled needs and unsatisfied demands.

(b) Change in the relative social status of men and women.
This has been another rapid and far-reaching change, again associated with culture-lag, in that many husbands and wives have

not yet satisfactorily assimilated the changed pattern. The conflict here may be between the two of them; but just as often it appears within each individual, who discovers contradictory motives within himself or herself, with conflicting social and political pressures adding to the confusion.

(c) Cultural differences in mate choice.
In itself this is sometimes a reaction to the incest taboo within the emotionally overcharged and insecurely possessive family of origin, implying a search for someone essentially different. Yet it is from this family of origin that the in-built models of a desired person must in any case arise, and these determine subsequent marital behaviour patterns, within the self and expected from the other. So where the original families are widely different, conflict becomes virtually inevitable, although not necessarily pernicious. Conflicts due to discrepancies in role patterns are very often denied at first, and may be repressed and avoided for a remarkably long time. For example, during the first five years or so of a marriage, personal relationship in any depth is often bypassed or 'postponed' because of urgent preoccupation with biological drives – sexual needs, home-building and caring for young children. Dicks refers to these preoccupations as 'subpersonal' rather than personal as far as the dyadic relationship is concerned; and it is often only after this phase that a couple begins to take stock of each other, and notice their short-comings as a pair. But when the need for deeper ways of relating increases, communication failures also increase. Awareness of this sad fact then tends to be fended off by continuing a collusive process of mutual idealisation, which may succeed in masking ambivalences, at least for a time. Excessive culture distance between the partners can be an important social factor in the breakdown of an insecure marriage propped up by idealisation.

The pressure towards autonomy and independence of young people characteristic of modern Western society not unexpectedly meets a resistance, coming from within the individual and from society itself, springing from the older, more secure order handed down by the culture-lag of generations. In this social conflict there is bound to be a certain proportion of people who will fail to adapt to the more challenging, much less structured demands of marital roles.

We come now to the *individual setting* in which conflict may arise. We have emphasised that there has been a transition from the patriarchal heteronomy of the traditional extended family to the present-day requirement of autonomy facing young adults who are getting married. We saw this really means that all the resources required for making satisfactory emotional commitments have to be carried inside the person as potential spouse, without the aid of unambiguous, authoritative directives, or strong group support. This requirement of autonomy presupposes an unprecedented achievement in overcoming emotional dependence on the family of origin. In his psychopathology, Dicks has always stressed the nuclear importance of infantile dependence as the starting-point of the capacity to make relationships (following Hadfield and Fairbairn) and its frustration as the beginning of neurosis. Success in marriage seems to require a blend of autonomy (implying secure personal identity and ego-strength) and the capacity for what Fairbairn called 'mature dependence'. In the event, the dependency needs have often *not* matured, but are instead split off in the self and denied, as a result of insecurity in the family of origin; and hence they have become a part of the personality that is repressed and lost to the self. Time and again we find that it is this split-off aspect of the self that the pseudo-independent young adult perceives in the partner, who then attracts because seeming to promise a re-discovery of that lost part of his own personality. We used the term 'projective identification' (Klein) to describe this; and it is often a mutual process, echoed in such phrases as 'you are part of me', 'I know you perfectly', and the like.

What is needed for a healthy marriage is a flexible readiness in both partners to adapt their mutual behaviour in response to each other's changing needs – the one being dependent, the other strong; then the other way round. This role flexibility amounts to the capacity to tolerate, 'fuse' and use ambivalence. The word 'fuse' implies the holding of love and hate together, 'containing' each other, not split into separate good and bad object-relations. Dick remarks that this is perhaps the key to the secret of all human relationships. The conflict of ambivalence comes at the time when the infant first becomes aware that his object is a separate person from himself. Later the objects become internalised. It is hoped that the ambivalence is fused (i.e. the bad tolerated by predominantly good experience), but instead it is often split and repressed. This situation has been studied intensively by Fairbairn, and a brief reference to his analysis might help understanding. It is inevitable that a small child's needs will at times be disapproved of and rejected by one or both of his parents. If this happens repeatedly, he may give up protesting and try to deny his needs. That is, he gives up on the real relationship with mother or father and tries to deal with his needs within his own mind. He 'introjects' the unfulfilling relationship, making an internal 'working model' of it (Bowlby) that persists alongside his day-to-day life with his actual parent. In this way he splits off the unsatisfying, worrying aspects of the parent from the real person, whom he is then more able to tolerate. He learns to disregard or 'repress' the needy part of himself (which Fairbairn calls the 'libidinal ego') – but more than that, he forms a model in his mind of the 'forbidding-rejecting-mother/father-refusing-to-accept-his-needs'. This is the 'antilibidinal object' in Fairbairn's terminology. As time goes on, he learns to live with his mother or father adequately in everyday life. The inner model of his 'desired-object-rejecting-his-needs' is bypassed in his psychic development, out of the main line of his growth – but it does not cease to exist. This is what is meant by the object-relation being 'split off', or 'repressed'. Later, in close relationship such as marriage, when he is again in a situation of responding instinctually to a close, exciting personal object, he does so on the basis of this pre-existing relational model – i.e. with an expectation of rejection, and hence hostility as well as desire. Thus the ambivalence becomes de-fused, with love switching suddenly into hate. This situation is often mutual and collusive, and in marital therapy there is frequently real difficulty in clarifying the boundaries between (i) parts of the ego, (ii) external object, and (iii) the internal object of fantasy in mutual interaction.

We are now coming into the area of *unconscious needs* of the third sub-system. If there is an inadequate sense of identity and ego-strength, the threat posed by defusion of ambivalent feelings can be too disruptive, and these tend to be held repressed. Hence the individual loses touch with his own ambivalent feelings, and by the same token is unable to tolerate the threat from his partner's either. Emotional freedom becomes unbearable, and a rigid defensive posture has to be adopted to preserve a brittle sense of selfhood based on the denial of 'badness' or demandingness. The same process is applied to the self and to the partner, who must conform to the taboo against being bad or demanding. The denial of the partner's ambivalence is attempted characteristically by using the cloak of idealisation. This is really a blocking of the ability to see him or her as a separate person distinct from the self, because accepting the true characteristics of the actual person would be too painful – e.g. too reminiscent of an uncaring, unsatisfying parent. There is an attempt, seldom if ever successfully sustained, to preserve the partner as a totally fulfilling figure – to the sacrifice of reality. He or she is coerced into the idealised role, identified with the subject's own need. This state of affairs is not at all stable, however, and is predictably accompanied by lapses into angry outbursts, bitter accusations and recriminations. When the process takes place reciprocally in both partners simultaneously (as it usually does) we have a collusion in which each invests part of himself in the other. There is a 'blurring of ego boundaries', as Dicks calls it: a fluidity and lack of clear demarcation between the two. Each may use the same

52

accusations against the other, and feel the same persecution from the other; and the 'symptoms' get passed between them, from one to the other. We feel we are in the presence of a joint dyadic ego; and in the shared feelings and objects we see the essential collusion that closely binds the disturbed marital dyad and presents the characteristic therapeutic problem. This unconsciously established complementariness accounts for the observation that couples who behave like cat-and-dog often have a deep sense of ownership and belonging; and it adds validity to such expressions as 'my other half'. This 'joint personality' enables each 'half' to *rediscover lost aspects of their own primary object-relations, which they can then re-experience by projective identification.* Dicks adheres strongly to the object-relations theory of Fairbairn and Guntrip, viz. that it is not 'feelings' or 'impulses' that are repressed, but *affective relationships that are split off* from the conscious self. This can happen at any of the significant developmental levels. E.g. (a) Klein's 'paranoid position' – angry oral frustration, with dread of loss of the *only* source of life and satisfaction of need. The chief feelings here are a deep mistrust, suspicion and possessive jealousy. (b) The 'depressive position' – characteristically ambivalent, with the need to preserve the object as good, so that the badness is all taken into the self. Here we get the attitudes of contrition and self-abasement, with restitutive behaviour. There is identification with the frustrating antilibidinal ego and inhibition of sexuality. At this level, marriage can appear as a defence against sexuality! (c) The 'schizoid position' is where withdrawal or obsessional detachment produces a sense of hollowness and doubt, with a cerebral effort to act out the loving role which is not experienced spontaneously. (d) 'Hysterical dissociation': this can give rise to functional disabilities such as impotence and frigidity.

With all these forms of relational disturbance and fragmentation there goes a deep fear of commitment – of giving oneself into the hands of another person. Hence one of the main results of the marital relationship initially is seen to be the defence of the insecure ego in the face of the stimulated primitive libidinal needs and fears.

We have perhaps covered enough ground now to understand the two main hypotheses that Dicks used to guide him in systematising his work.

Hypothesis (1) was as follows. Many tensions between partners seem to result from the disappointment which one or both feel when the other fails to play the role expected, after the manner of a preconceived model or figure in their fantasy world – usually a desired parental model, or a contrast to a parental model. This relates to the failure of idealisation, threatening the resurgence of ambivalence. Later he added a rider to this hypothesis, stating that tensions between partners can result from disappointment that the partner does, after all, play the marital role *just like the original frustrating parent figure*, similarity to whom was earlier denied. This discovery (often collusive) leads to the subject then changing his own behaviour to a more childish, so-called 'regressed' pattern, in response to his perception of the partner as a dominating parent.

Hypothesis (2) stated that subjects may persecute in their spouses tendencies which originally caused attraction when the partner was perceived unconsciously as if he were a lost (because actually split-off) part of the subject's own personality. This refers to the process of projective identification. This was mentioned earlier, but a further brief explanation might be helpful. The individual senses some aspect of the partner to which he feels powerfully drawn. He is not at the time fully aware, if at all, that he is seeing in the partner some quality he *recognises*, because it belongs to him, as it were. It represents a forgotten part of himself that is still seeking recognition. So he projects this part of himself into the partner whom he then treats as the personification of his unrecognised self – i.e. he identifies the partner with himself. Later reality-testing shows how mistaken he is. Then, instead of cherishing the partner as his own needy child aspect, he sees only the hard reality of his partner *being* needy and making demands of him – an intolerable circumstance for him, always tending to provoke bitter rage.

With increasing experience in the study of cases, degrees of interaction were observed that in depth and complexity went beyond the scope of these original hypotheses. Conflict in marriage seems to become overriding when the unifying forces of biological impulsion, everyday reality and adult social norms have lost their holding power, and the ultimate refuge of idealisation has failed. Then we see the appearance of ambivalence and its defusion – the upsurge of primitive, essentially contradictory and unfulfillable object-needs towards each other, expressed in paradoxical, heavily disguised, oblique ways – love expressed by sulks, revenge, angry provocation – in short, by every device of 'representation by the opposite'. The picture becomes one of infantile love-and-hate interaction, in which the central egos of the participants are relatively powerless (although functioning usually quite normally outside the marriage). The marital dyad is now reproducing the conflicts over regressive attempts to recapture the desired gratifications of the symbiotic primary relationship of infant and mother. Dicks states that the marital bonds, both in health and disease, are the nearest adult equivalent to the original primary parent-child relation. Projective identification, so prominent in marital dyad transactions, belongs to the primary infant level – the schizoid, or pre-depressive, position. The primary projective bonds, which represent an attempt to deal with ambivalence by splitting, and in essence constitute a simple paranoid mechanism, are the essential ones in the dyadic conflicts. 'The less well the individual has been able to sort out his first phase of development, the more these inner structures remain fully charged, and at the slightest provocation we have regressive behaviour' (Teruel). In the dyad, such regression becomes an interpenetration, through mutual projections, of the private inner worlds of both partners, so that ultimately their shared private worlds become more and more common property between them.

When they are shared completely we have a 'folie à deux'.

So out of the original hypotheses we have a picture in greater depth of marital conflict, involving the activation of many and changing projections and re-projections, forming a complex system of conflicting yet shared object-relational needs and drives at a very primitive level. This happens in the attempt to solve each individual's own inner contradictions through the partner, while still maintaining the dyadic integrity necessary to achieve this. In the collusion that occurs, each in the first instance seeks to protect his own libidinal ego from his introjected anti-libidinal object which may now be re-projected into the spouse. Secondly, they collude in defending the joint 'social personality' they have created in marrying each other. In publicly defending the partner whom he or she persecutes, each is secretly cherishing that 'bad' aspect of self that he or she has projected into the partner. Dicks maintains that the collusive marriage, in which internal persecuting objects are shared and polarised in this dialectic fashion, may be said to represent the closest approximation we have to the intra-personal resolution of conflict: a view of marriage as 'natural' psychotherapy! In his book, he quotes many meticulously observed and detailed case studies to illustrate how his concepts were arrived at, and he presents his evidence convincingly. He concludes the section on marital psychopathology with a comment on the interaction of his three sub-systems. This helps to explain certain recurrent patterns in *dyadic adaptation* to the ambivalent investment of the partners – which is what he means by 'marital tensions'. This condition of adaptation, or dyadic homeostasis, designed to maintain the stability of the relationship, depends on each partner's ability to deal with the pressure in the third sub-system (their unconscious interactions) in one of the following ways:

    (a) By congruence of all three subsystems, i.e. the perception of each other as whole, separate persons, with negotiated 'benign' conflict resolution.

(b) By using shared cultural and personal (conscious) norms as *defences* against impulsion from the libidinal/anti-libidinal (unconscious) object-relation levels. This is collusive defence: by idealisation, convention, 'rationality', moral consensus, etc. Conflict is not allowed to appear openly, is denied, or explained away.

(c) By the collusive *using of these shared norms as a façade* behind which the object-relational problems are *acted out* by means of projective and introjective mechanisms, the needs inherent in these problems being shared. This situation may follow the nature of (b). The resulting interaction appears as a paranoid or depressive dyadic system, in which the expression of anger or hate often seems more satisfying than love. The first and second subsystems are maintained in public, to keep peace with the outside world (which becomes the repository of peace and stability) and to support the arena where the domestic conflict is being conducted.

Finally Dicks refers to the failed marriage which breaks up. A marriage may prove unviable at any of the three levels: but in his view it would seem necessary for at least two of the three subsystems to function satisfactorily if the dyad is to survive – e.g. social affinity + congruence of deep object-relations can withstand strong divergences of personal norms and tastes, etc. But if reality-testing shows that there is nothing but social affinity, or shared interests, or seeing only a good parent or exciting lover to offset loneliness, then the marriage will sooner or later be dead. 'The opposite of love, he concludes, 'is not hate. These two always co-exist as long as there is a live relationship. The opposite to love is indifference.'

Henry V Dicks   Marital Tensions: Clinical Studies Towards a Psychological Theory of Interaction (First published 1967)

List of researchers:

Bowlby, John
Fairbairn, Ronald
Guntrip, Harry
Hadfield, J A
Klein, Melanie
Teruel, Guillermo

Marital Therapy in Action

In this paper I wish to present a particular view of marital therapy, relating it to the study of a case that I have created, using situations and dynamics that are not uncommon in martial problems. This paper was originally a lecture that arose out of work in a psychiatric clinic – hence the medical terminology, which I no longer believe to be satisfactory, e.g. the use of the words 'patient', 'illness' etc.

My interest in this subject arose out of making one or two very simple observations familiar to everybody who has watched patients and their spouses in different situations. For example:

1) One notices that often the spouse, when seen, appears surprisingly different from the person expected from having listened to the patient's account. Similarly, a married couple seen together may behave in a way that contradicts their behaviour when seen separately, often to an arresting degree.

2) I was struck by the well known fact that married couples could make each other so consistently unhappy, yet stick together and strongly resist any pressure to separate.

3) I was surprised to note how often the spouse did not at all welcome what to me seemed a gratifying improvement in the patient's mental health. I had one egocentric obsessional man, whose docile and anxious wife became more confident. He complained that she was 'getting *far too well!*'

4) I had noticed that successful treatment, or remission, of mental illness was sometimes associated with growth of disturbance in the mental health of the spouse, as if the

focus of disability in a 'sick marriage' could be transferred from one partner to the other.

5) Recently I had a case where a depressed patient was divorced by his wife, whereupon *she* suffered from an acute psychotic episode.

6) It seemed that all this linked up with the well known finding that, in families, the person who asks for help in the role of patient can be, at the time, the least disturbed member; and soon after the initial referral, the emphasis shifts to another member or members.

7) One of the most familiar observations of all springs to mind in this context, namely that behaviour disorders in children draw attention to the disturbed relationship in their parents' marriage – of which they are usually a symptom.

These simple observations made me want to look more closely at the marital dyad. This would be the point to quote Harry Stack Sullivan's definition of psychiatry as 'the operational statement of interpersonal relations', because here it was the *relation* that was disturbed rather than one or other of the separate elements. Here too one wants to mention the psychodynamics of Fairbairn, with its emphasis on the subject-object bond as the essential element, rather than the Freudian preoccupation with 'impulses' inherent in the subject. With Fairbairn's model of personality functioning we surely have a natural paradigm in the marital dyad, with the 'self' seeking support in the object. An obvious concept, one might think, for the understanding and treatment of neurosis.

The location of symptomatology *in the relationship alone* is seen most clearly in those cases presenting as a couple with problems, although this is not the commonest group who come for help. Couples who present themselves together often see 'the illness', so-called, in their partner, and separately they do not complain of symptoms at all – except that they are unhappy, of course. Separately they may cope perfectly well. Typically in this group the psychiatric abnormality appears clearly to be a part of their relationship together, at the interface, as it were, of their contact within that relationship. Away from this meeting point they appear as persons who, although unhappy, are not mentally 'sick' in any sense; and if they do consult us separately, it is usually to draw attention to the relationship. E.g. 'I have been so depressed because of him.' 'If only she could be different...' and so on.

The commonest way in which cases are referred to us, however, is that of the individual patient with symptoms. He or she comes from the hospital outpatient department or from an inpatient ward, with some psychoneurotic or character disorder for which psychotherapy seems to be indicated. If in our assessment it seems to be that marriage figures significantly (and I have been impressed by how often this does reflect the problem to an important degree), a joint interview involving the spouse would be arranged, and their interaction observed with several questions in mind:

- Is there a dyad, i.e. a viable ongoing relationship, good or bad?
- What sort of communication exists between them?
- What, if any, motivation for change seems to be present?

Perhaps we can then observe obvious areas of conflict that could be usefully explored.

If it appears that the couple are having difficulties with a real libidinal involvement and not attempting to flog a dead horse, we might then decide upon marital therapy, with or without simultaneous treatment of one or other spouse in another therapeutic situation. The couple would then be seen separately, and a personal history, including their personal view of the problem, would be obtained. Sometimes, indeed more often than not, the history of the spouse shows up a psychopathology complementary in significant ways to that of the nominal patient. After these preliminary investigations, the couple would be invited to attend a series of joint interviews with two therapists, a male and a female, usually at two-weekly intervals. This choice of the 'foursome' as an interview method has a number of advantages which should emerge clearly as we discuss cases. Our initial preference arose from the need to minimise the risk of 'taking sides', and to have an observer of one's own involvement. What happens in this process can best be told by describing a case such as the one I have created below.

Bill and Maureen are in their late twenties. They have been married for 6 years. To all appearances they are a pleasant, ordinary couple with a good home and two young children. Neither suffered any psychiatric disturbance whatever until the beginning of the fourth year of their marriage, when Bill complained to his GP of symptoms diagnosed as 'anxiety and depression'. This began when their house, in which they had invested a good deal in improvements, was threatened with demolition because of pipe-laying underneath. Apart from the obvious cause for worry, the symbolic significance of this situation did not escape us.

Bill had three spells of hospital treatment in two and a half years, but with little or no effect. He continued to feel depressed and depersonalised, lacked confidence and became increasingly unhappy at home. Maureen says he became a 'nervous wreck', and that there had been no happiness in the home for the past three of their six married years. During his last admission he complained mainly of his marital difficulties, viz. – *Thinking only about himself and his discontents; not bothering about wife and children. At times having no feeling at all for them. Upsetting his wife. At times she admitted having no feelings for him, and she got depressed herself, feeling that he was no use as a husband and she felt like leaving him. He felt he didn't care; but at other times he worried desperately that his marriage was breaking up. Formerly obsessionally conscientious, he felt he now wanted to run away from his responsibilities. Each upset the other, and they quarrelled incessantly, sometimes separating for a few days, but soon coming together again.*

After Bill's third spell of hospital treatment they were referred to us as a couple at the Psychotherapy Unit. We have seen each separately once, and have had six joint sessions to date in foursome-type interviews with a female nurse and myself. The following gives a sketch of their backgrounds:

Bill is the eldest of three children. His father, a HGV driver, is a heavy drinker; a rough and ready, superficially outgoing man, tough, but popular with his cronies. But aside from his outward sociability, Bill says his father is really a lonely man, who has been understanding with him in his recent troubles. At home he can be loudly argumentative when drinking. Bill's mother, unlike her husband, seems to be rather isolated and rarely goes out socially. She presents herself as being devoted to her children, and has tended to indulge Bill. She seems to have tried to keep his affection this way. He always thought she was a 'great mother', but he never *felt* as close to her as to his father. During Bill's second hospital admission (a year after the first) it was noted: *Contrary to his first description of his family, he is now greatly troubled by his feelings towards his mother. 'She is a right hard bitch, but she puts on a soft and good front... It's all a front. My father seems a bit rough, but he does seem to understand.'* Bill told us that his mother rather despises his father, and has caused him personal embarrassment by saying she 'prefers him'. He used to think his family was 'perfect'. His acknowledgement of the shadow side came during the period when marital problems came to the forefront at the time of his second admission to hospital.

Maureen is the eldest of numerous children. As far back as she can remember, there were always younger children to look after, and she has always had to deputise for her mother, no matter what her own wishes were. She was well looked after materially, but feels she had too much responsibility. She thinks she got on quite well with her mother, but has the feeling that she can't trust her. 'She talks behind your back', despite seeming to mean well. As if to make some excuse for her, she told me that her mother had been an unloved child, brought up to be grateful. The family are Catholics. Maureen's father had disapproved of her marrying a

Protestant, yet despite this, she feels closer to him than to her mother. He is quite a heavy drinker. Mother never stressed his good points, and tended to present father in a bad light and herself in a good light. Father was from North America and has never felt settled in this country. He is a scaffolder, and it seems he has stayed over here to please mother. Maureen says 'He is like me, chicken-hearted, and ruled by my mother.' Maureen could never stand up for herself at home. She always did what she was told, yet often felt it was an unfair imposition. At home the family were never allowed to express their feelings. If they tried, it was regarded as cheek, and angrily reacted against by mother. Her parents hardly ever took Maureen into their confidence. One major event she cannot forgive them for is that they went on holiday to her father's former home without telling her, and missed her wedding.

At the time that Bill and Maureen married, Bill expected his wife to be someone who would look after him and be tolerant of him. He was happy to find that this was what Maureen set out to do to his satisfaction – until their first child was born, after which her attention was divided. For her part, Maureen saw her husband as big and strong – which he is, physically. 'Someone to lean on' as she put it, which was just what she wanted. But she soon found out that in fact he was usually quite unassertive and passive, and before long she was taking over and managing things. This 'just happened', and she was not aware of any disappointment at that time. In her account of Bill's 'illness', she saw it as a quite sudden change in a previously well balanced personality. For the three years before it, he had been very quiet, only exceptionally expressing annoyance. 'He was still a bachelor.' But since then he became more active and talkative. Maureen feels *she* may have brought about this change in him – a change she approves of, but one she feels guilty about in case it 'might have brought on his illness'. During the marriage, she too has changed, from being a soft, unforceful person to being the decisive, controlling one, taking all the responsibilities. She later admitted how resentful she felt about this. From Bill's viewpoint, however, he seemed to have found what he wanted – someone dependable, willing to care for him. He responded by trying to meet her wishes by being sociable and talkative, although his inclination was to be passive. Sometimes he showed his resentment about this, and then Maureen felt guilty. So by the time their first child was born, both of them were feeling disappointed and somewhat angry at the failure of their spouse to meet their original expectations. This became more overt in later interviews.

When his 'illness' began, Bill's lively manner at home disappeared and he became withdrawn and inert, lying about in bed, showing no interest in his wife or in the home, complaining of being depressed and 'shut off from life by a partition behind his eyes'. This last symptom (of depersonalisation), he noted, disappeared when he was involved in an aggressive game of football, which he continued to play. At home he became bad tempered and quarrelsome. At first Maureen reacted by becoming even more capable and coping, but soon grew less and less tolerant. When he went into hospital she was very tearful, but denied feeling angry. She felt frustrated at his inability to pull himself out of his depression, and she 'lost the ability to sympathise with him'. At times she had a panicky feeling that she had no feelings for him at all.

Throughout this period of illness it appeared that when Bill was most depressed and helpless, Maureen tended to be the strong coping one – often seeming to be quite hard and managing; but periodically she 'cracked up' and felt depressed herself, whereupon Bill took over in a 'tough' manner, sweeping her aside, 'as if he didn't care about her anyway'. At times he even left home in these circumstances, and went to his parent's house for a few days. This 'see-saw' phenomenon, in which the couple seemed to share the 'illness' reciprocally, became very clear in the early marital interviews.

Because Bill became the nominal 'patient', let us note briefly what was involved in his 'depressive illness':

On his second admission he was crying, saying that he didn't know whether he was coming or going. He said that he felt like a small child whereas he should feel like a man. At home he was unable to discuss things with his wife. He came home from work and fell asleep, and was then unable to sleep at night. He had nightmares in which people were chasing him to hurt him, and he was without refuge. He would wake up in a cold sweat. He considered that his wife was intolerant and hard, although he realised that he was contributing to her growing feelings of depression. He could understand when she said that they might have to separate. There had been numerous quarrels and he had felt like hitting her. The prospect of work was so depressing that he found it hard to get up. He felt that he was 'always angry', and that his anger was only just under control. He said that it would be 'terrible' if he lost control. He was angry with the hospital for 'sending him out too soon' last time. He said they were 'not interested in understanding him, but only in curing him' (*sic*). He had aggressive fantasies of killing himself with a knife.

This was more or less the situation when they began marital therapy. I will turn now to the kind of interviews that would take place. (My sample comments are in italics.)

Session 1
Bill was extremely passive, bland, and expressing no emotion whatever. He quietly repeated that the situation seemed to him to be hopeless, and that there was nothing he could do. Maureen became quite emotional, frequently burst into tears, and eventually admitted that she was very angry and felt like shaking him. I said *she seemed to be the one expressing all the feeling for both of them*. It transpired that Bill had manoeuvred his GP to be angry with his former therapist. When it was pointed out that *he got other people to express the anger he himself was feeling* he became restless, glared, and thereafter withdrew. Maureen said that her own angry criticism of him just drove him further into himself.

Session 2

This took place approximately a month later. Bill was more openly emotional than before, and Maureen was much less distressed. Bill said he had been surprised to find himself so assertive with his foreman at work, who had been imposing on him. Maureen said she wished he would show more of his feelings at home. She said it was a relief even when he was angry. What she could not bear was his withdrawal and apparent indifference. They spoke of his recent escapade of going to his parents for a week. Maureen taunted him that his doting mother sees no wrong in him, and no sooner does he run back than she is looking after him like a baby. This produced a flash of annoyance from Bill, who said that his mother's fussing made him feel rotten, and he had not been in the house five minutes before he wanted to leave again. Maureen then admitted her own bitter feeling about Bill's mother, who criticises her for not looking after him properly.

Session 3

At the third session, a few weeks later, Bill arrived alone. He said Maureen was too upset and depressed to come. He himself had left home once again and gone to his parents. He appeared quite calm, although he said he was worried about his lack of feeling for his wife. He didn't seem to care whether he went back or not. He felt okay at his parent's house. His father took the view that he should go home and finish the job he had taken on, but he didn't nag him. His mother disagreed and backed him up in his flight. He knew that this was because she disliked Maureen, and felt annoyed with himself for not asserting himself. *It was now his parents who were expressing the contradictory feeling about his marriage.* He was then able to discuss how divided he was within himself: on the one hand wanting to be cared for like a child, on the other hand feeling he really did want to take a stronger personal attitude. This led to discussion of his fear of authority, including that of doctors, and of his underlying resentment. (I did not remark upon the transference allusion.)

Session 4

A fortnight later it was Maureen's turn to come alone, very tearful and distressed. Bill was back at home again. She said 'Now *he* is quite calm and okay, and I'm all upset and can't cope.' It seemed Bill was now looking after the children, bathing them, feeding them, etc, because she felt too depressed and helpless. She said 'Anyway this is more like my real self', and that her former competence 'had just been a front'. I said that it *seemed now that Bill was wearing the coping front* and she agreed. When asked how she felt about this, she said she was afraid to say anything, or express any feeling in case she put him off, adding 'I do need support, although I pretended not to before.'

Session 5

At the next joint meeting, a week later, Maureen had regained her self-possession. Bill, too, appeared more equable. In this atmosphere, they proceeded to discuss their see-saw relationship. They saw that each wanted to lean on the other, and they took it in turns. The hard part was the bad temper that seemed to go with it. They spoke of their mutual expectations of each other when first married, and noted the fact that they were practically the same: i.e. wanting someone trustworthy to lean on. They also discussed their family backgrounds, particularly criticising their mothers. I said *it seemed they had both been searching for a missing 'good' relationship with mother when they came to get married.* Both of them said, in effect, yes, but sadly they had disappointed each other.

Session 6

This meeting took place a few weeks later. The couple began by saying that they were getting on better. Almost immediately, however, Bill qualified this by saying he 'still lacked feeling' for his wife and children. Maureen then began to cry. I said I felt that they were *both a bit angry, perhaps, below the surface, but found this difficult to admit in case they upset things again.* Then

68

Maureen turned on Bill and said 'No wonder – because he would never allow me to depend on him! Why couldn't he be a proper husband?' Bill blandly agreed that was how it was. Maureen then became furious, and turned to us, weeping loudly, saying she couldn't even be allowed to feel justified in being angry. 'He just agrees, and says he can't help it!' Bill agreed (again) that he just accepts criticism and then often does nothing about it. We said that *this was just a way of undermining Maureen's anger, and not acceptance at all.* Bill tried to get into a discussion with me about what he 'ought to do' about his behaviour. I said that one of his problems was his tendency to *get someone to tell him what to do,* and brought it back to himself and Maureen. They spoke of their attempts to manoeuvre each other to satisfy their wants, and their reluctance to talk about this openly because of a fear of angry reaction. I said it seemed that *each wanted the other to be the angry one; and neither wanted to admit being partly at fault, and having to change, rather than attempting to make the other one change.*

Session 7

At the next session their angry disappointment came into the open. Maureen wept and stamped with rage, accusing Bill of being utterly self-centred, sorry for himself, expecting her to sympathise endlessly, etc. For the first time in a joint session Bill was also openly angry, and shouted that she never bloody well noticed when he *did* show concerns. He had been trying to do something about his faults, but what was the use? He could never get through to her. Here his rage subsided into tears. He said Maureen had no interest in him as he was, but continually criticised and was discontented with him. A lot she said was only too true, he admitted, but he couldn't bear being continually put down as a washout. He wept quite bitterly. I said it seemed *they both felt persecuted and rejected, each by the other – as if each had a picture of the other being cold and angry.* When I made this comment, they were both in tears, and for the first time they

69

seemed to be sharing the feeling of frustrated dependency, which previously they had acted out separately in their reciprocal 'see-saw' way. Maureen then began to talk about her mother, whom she was always trying to please, as if she had to prove to her mother that she really cared about her. These efforts never seemed to succeed, and she never felt that her mother understood. Her sister was more successful, and more attractive, and was the favourite. Maureen had never got over the miserable feeling that her mother wasn't really interested in her. Bill came in here, and criticised her sister angrily, supporting Maureen. Then he said he too 'had always known that his mother never really cared a rap for him in spite of all her talk'. It was his father he felt like crying for in this bloody mess. Maureen confirmed that his mother seemed to care only for herself and her own ideas, and seemed to have no real relationship with him at all. Bill said nobody really helped; and he often felt annoyed with us, as if we were not helping him either. Both of them then said they sometimes felt it was no use coming here, and it was just a waste of time. At the end of the meeting they spoke of the fear they had of finding that maybe they didn't love each other after all, and this time they were sharing this anxiety.

[This seemed to me to be a crucial point in our meetings. The couple had allied together in their feeling of rejection, and were supporting each other against the cold, uncaring mother, *external to their relationship*, which they felt they shared. They exchanged handkerchiefs for their tears, and appeared to find comfort in each other's presence. This feeling of mutual support in their misery persisted. They were even discussing the doubts they had about their own feelings for each other, instead of attacking the other for having no feelings. This seemed to indicate that the projected bad persecuting object they shared had been taken back inside. Up to this point, this meeting showed that the couple shared a bad internal object, which each had projected into the spouse, and then felt attacked by. The object here appeared as the antilibidinal mother, possessive and rejecting.]

70

Maureen also spoke about her young brother who had just left home to seek his fortune. She wept as she said she was worried about him. Bill dryly interjected 'He can look after himself fine!' Maureen said she felt a desire to be with him, in case he got hurt. *I said she seemed to be describing in her brother the sort of vulnerable, needy person that Bill had usually appeared to be, and that she was perhaps describing another aspect of her feelings for Bill – a protective desire to shield him: to treat him as if he were helpless.* She admitted she did feel like this often, and 'knowing what it was like herself, she was terribly sorry for Bill', despite being so angry.

[Here Maureen acknowledged her own intense dependent need, and her attempt to deal with it in Bill by *being* the good mother. This demonstrated how projective identification complicated her relationship with Bill. Her helpless dependent self was perceived in him; and in so far as she identified with the helpless child in Bill, she encouraged him to remain dependent so that she could succour him, and relieve her own distress – which she was perceiving in him. Yet at the same time, she was hating him for his dependent demands and lack of adult concern. So she was actually *colluding unconsciously* in sustaining the very aspects of Bill that she consciously attacked. This perhaps accounts for her feelings of guilt that she had 'maybe made him the way he was'.]

Although certain aspects of psychopathology have been demonstrated in 'session 7', this would not necessarily mean that the situation between Bill and Maureen, and with us, was fully clarified. Yet I think that I have showed quite plainly some of the processes that, for example, Henry Dicks describes in his treatise 'Marital Tensions'; and these processes do seem to operate in many marriage problems. The patients usually come into marriage, like Bill and Maureen, as 'needy' individuals whose personalities are still bound up with ambivalent, unstable internal object-relations. During the courtship, the 'bad' side of the partner's character tends to be denied, and irrational expectations of love-fulfilment and shared 'goodness' are kept alive by the maintenance of a mutual idealisation. When this breaks down, the hostility that always underlies idealisation emerges. The romance ends, and the partner appears as a let-down and a disappointment. As often as not, only the bad, frustrating elements seem to be left, from which (as with all ambivalence) there seems to be no escape. In our case, the threat to the couple then was depression – loss of the ideal good mother. This was only inadequately countered by their projections and denials.

This situation of unfulfilled ideal expectations, leading to angry rejection that becomes reciprocal, is one of the simplest and maybe the most characteristic of marital problems for which guidance is sought. Some couples are able to work through this situation surprisingly quickly to reach a better level of tolerance and understanding of each other. All that seems to be required is the presence of the accepting 'neutral' therapists who can resist pressures to take sides, and can assist the couple's mutual communication. With other couples, the failure of mutual ideal expectations seems to act as a detonator that sets off a series of deeper events, involving unconscious needs of both personalities that are reciprocal and intertwining, so that the resultant interaction becomes more and more binding and collusive. This is what appeared to occur in the example I have drawn up. Looking at this interaction in marital therapy, it appears as a set of co-existent but split-off fragmentary relationships, or in Fairbairn's language, the 'partial egos' of a dyad, bound up in relation to shared objects, in which the ego boundaries of the partners have become blurred by partial absorption each within the other. These partial relationships date back to the early historical experiences of both partners, as can often be seen clearly enough. What makes the situation a significant treatment problem is its collusive quality that makes the spouses need each other in this morbid way, despite their manifest problems.

The breakthrough in treatment comes through the mediation of transference, although perhaps not in the usual sense. In many examples, this takes a simple form that does not require extensive analysis. It is as if we are present as the custodians of the adult aspects of the couple – their good sense, supportiveness and willingness to help – aspects that between themselves become swamped by their infantile struggles with their shared object-relations. Provided they can allow their otherwise repressed adult supportiveness to reside in us, they will allow us to intervene helpfully about unwelcome aspects of their relationship, normally concealed by fear, quarrelling and recrimination. Since this is accepted as helpful by them both, and we are experienced as supportive, it is possible to (a) help them to tolerate their own 'badness' without feeling destructively persecuted by the other; and (b) enable them to discover their own, more adult, supportive selves, which they can then take back from us. They can then *help each other* to work through their day-to-day difficulties.

This seems to me to be the essential core of marital therapy as such. In some cases, that is as far as the therapeutic intervention goes, and there is a quick, positive improvement.

I now produce an example of this by creating a young couple, married for three years, where the wife presented with a florid hysterical upset at home – tears, depression, whining infantile behaviour, petulant silence and frigidity – yet without apparently any disturbance whatever in her work. Her husband was calm, capable and managing, very emotionally detached, and treated her as a patient when we saw them. The girl was re-enacting an experience of abandonment by mother in infancy, and her upbringing by aloof foster parents. By his 'professional' management of her, the husband played the part of the foster parents, while at the same time denying his own anger, disappointment and distress – which she expressed, and with which he at once projectively identified. Once again we have the situation where each member of the dyad maintains the other, unconsciously, in the morbid role which consciously they complain of.

The crux of the therapy was a session in which the wife had a very angry outburst, accusing her husband of unreliability and pettiness, little deceits and inadequacies under his competent façade. He had to admit this, supported by our acceptance. Later, he spoke of his fears and of his distress; and this allowed his wife to move into a more adult position. At their last meeting, this couple had no symptoms, appeared much happier and were cooperating successfully together.

Here our intervention was limited to helping the couple out of the fixed, extreme positions they were defensively maintaining that were reducing their marriage to a travesty of psychiatric nursing. The deeper individual reasons for the neurotic behaviour were not fully explored by us. This did not seem necessary. Our aim was not to bring about radical personality change, but to help to start them off, hoping that, in time, they would do it themselves. We aimed to release the dyad from a restrictive neurotic formation which they were maintaining in collusion – the pattern of marriage as a 'nursing' problem. You will remember that Bill and Maureen colluded in maintaining the pattern of marriage as a battle.

Bill and Maureen's collusive system was based on *sharing* a rejecting mother. This last 'case' had a system based on *polarisation*, where one became the helpless child-patient while the other had to become the omnipotent parent-nurse. We could see how the couple had each other trapped in a binding infantile relation; and identifying these systems enabled treatment to focus quickly upon the aspect of interaction where resistance was centred. They tried to deal with their depression by passing it from one to the other like a hot brick. The other couple dealt with their terrifying helplessness by freezing into fixed roles. But neither couple presented us with a united front of resistance, because the negative transference, as it were, was tied up in their dyadic relation. In both cases we maintained a useful degree of positive contact that reassured them both.

Another kind of case is that in which the introjected hostile object is projected into the therapists, and the typical negative transference does emerge in therapy. Treatment of this kind of situation may lead to rapid improvement, too, although it is not unlikely to involve the couple joining forces in attacking the therapist instead of each other. What we have found in this event illustrates another advantage of the two-therapist interview, in that it is usually only one of the therapists who is attacked, while the other is allowed to be supportive and maintain positive contact. Provided the therapists can cope with this stress successfully, the situation can again be worked through as before.

There are many other cases, however, in which the transference situation is more complex: for example, where therapists as well as spouses become involved as primitive part-objects. But that must remain another story!

Summary of dynamics:

1) Failure of ideal expectations.
   (Henry Dick's 'Hypothesis 1')
2) Appearance of ambivalence and threat of depression.
3) Failure of denial defences and onset of depression.
4) Marital defences: Collusive projective identification –
   (a) Collusion in sharing the bad object – the 'see-saw'.
   (b) Collusion in polarisation of fixed roles.

List of researchers:

Dicks, Henry V   'Marital Tensions'
Fairbairn, Ronald
Sullivan, Harry Stack

How are we to talk about people?
Is there a common language of the person?

This is the last lecture given by Dr Taylor before he retired from the NHS in the early 1980s.

A major problem in writing and speaking about persons, and personal encounters such as psychotherapy and counselling, is how to prevent our words from getting between ourselves and the actual life-situation. Somehow we must ensure that we do not end up with *ideas about* the person rather than knowledge of his real being. If the error of science is to dissect the person out of existence, the existentialist error is to lose him in concepts of totality. These are two extremes that overlook the fact that the person is not only real and meaningful in himself, but is also, in a simple direct and ordinary way, real and meaningful to us *in our own experience*, as we encounter him in life. It is to this fact that we should perhaps be addressing ourselves. This must involve acceptance of the limitations of definition and conceptualisation, i.e. theory-making, and it throws us back on our own personal resources, such as they are, in an attempt to discover what is most meaningful in the encounter. This is the essence of my argument.

So how *do* we talk about people? The deeper question is how do we experience ourselves in relation to people, and can we reach through to their experience of each other and of us?

We are all persons sharing the same world, and our life involves a common concern. To be human, we must not only understand but must also care about each other. Indeed it is becoming more and more obvious that to survive at all in an increasingly dangerous world we must even love one another. Yet we are taught not to. We are conditioned to compete, and to succeed at other people's expense; to seek and wield power; to exploit and coerce people; to be self-seeking. J Henry (quoted in R D Laing's 'The Politics of Experience') wrote: 'In a society where competition for the basic cultural goods is a pivot of action, people cannot be taught to love one another. It thus becomes necessary for the school to teach children how to hate; and without appearing to do so, for our culture cannot tolerate the idea that babes should hate each other.' This is an appalling truth about the antithesis of caring. We ignore it at our peril. It reminds us that we are led to regard people simply as factors in our environment, to be adapted to, controlled or mastered, as we have done with the natural world. From this standpoint, people become things.

From caring to technology

My standpoint is that of a doctor who chose to become a psychotherapist. In our current epoch, medicine comes under the aegis of science, whose enormous success in extending man's power over nature has led it to dominate almost all our thinking. The 'in' thing is for doctors and psychiatrists to be scientific, virtually at all costs. It was not always so. Medicine was a caring art long before science won over our minds. In many important ways it fortunately still is. But the pressure exerted all through one's psychiatric training and practice is to remember one's medical background and think scientifically about the mind – which, after all, one is told, is only an index of what is 'really' happening in the brain. This prejudice acts at once to isolate me within a particular professional clique set apart from those of a different professional calling who are equally concerned with healing human anguish. Worse than that, it not only splits me off from others whose work seems parallel to my own, but also ties me into a system (the medical-scientific system) which is actually quite ill-suited to my aims. My aims are all to do with meeting and understanding *persons*, with communicating about persons and with the language of common human experience. Natural science has little or nothing to tell me about these matters. Nor has modern medicine. Although it can be said that doctors care for human beings, these words are ambiguous. 'Care' is a primal word with antithetical meanings. It can mean the burden life lays upon one; it can mean the relieving of that burden; it can mean being concerned; and it can mean a nurturing relationship that fosters growth. Doctors are becoming less and less willing to share the burdens of their patients. The trend is to become less and less personally concerned. Although as a result of medical work suffering and ill-health have obviously been greatly relieved, the unmistakeable tendency is to drift away from caring and into technology. The personal care of former times, when medical science was so helpless, has been replaced by clever but impersonal techniques and amazing machines. Psychotherapy must take note of this, because it is, in my view, the parting of the ways. The Self cannot be accounted for by scientific reductionism. The ultimate meaningful entity which we know as the 'person' cannot be reduced to physico-chemical processes any more that Monet's 'Waterlilies' can be explained by the chemistry of pigment or the physiology of perception. The very essence of the matter disappears in the attempt. Dr J D Sutherland once said: 'In facing reductionist beliefs we must ask ourselves is anything more real to us than our Self as a free agent?' Yet because of the immense influence of scientific determination, the simple, ordinary experience of the reality of self has come to be overlooked, doubted, disparaged and even denied to an amazing extent. In so far as the psychotherapist sees the Self as the centre of his interest, he has parted company with modern medicine.

If we glance at how doctors talk about people, we see the doctor as the expert who 'knows' (the teacher); and the person facing him professionally is reduced to the subordinate position of 'the patient' (the passive sufferer) who submits to being treated. There is no way that psychotherapy as I understand it could proceed along these lines. I would consider my objective to be enabling a person to win his freedom to *be* a person, and (the other aspect of freedom) the acceptance of personal responsibility. And surely he can achieve this only through the experience of his *equality* with me: the exact opposite of treating him as a patient upon whom health has to be conferred by expertise. So, when working within a 'health service' I had to spend time with people restructuring our relationship to get rid of the doctor-patient idea – and not always to their liking I might say, as many hankered after the miracles that they had learned to expect from (of course) science!

The centrality of the person

It depresses me that so many academic psychologists get bogged down in their materialistic minutiae and never arrive at the person. Some do set out to get to know people, but usually in the mass, so that the person becomes a statistical abstraction. It is sad for me to look across the gulf that separates me from those other carers, such as pastors, social workers and others who may have been less blinded by science. I imagine them as probably less prone to the errors of reductionism, and, I hope, less corrupted by technology and techniques. But they may be tempted. The danger is all-pervasive and they must be vigilant. Everything we do can so easily become institutionalised and deteriorate into an unreflecting technique. Certainly psychotherapy has suffered from the disease of technique. In the textbooks it has its 'prescribed procedures'. And yet the most constant factor in outcome studies is that improvement is far less related to technique than to the interest and genuine concern of the therapist. How remarkable! But it had to be proved scientifically! Technique eventually dulls interest, and when rigorously practised becomes boring. This fact should be noted.

I feel certain that the model for psychotherapy cannot be that of an elitist, highly-specialised technical skill. I think that it is in fact just the opposite. I think that the model should derive from the experience of ordinary everyday life, from which the distressed person has become alienated, and back to which he will return if our help succeeds. I believe that psychotherapy should be an extension of our natural human reaction to a distressed person; and this is not a form of 'scientific discipline'. The prototype is perhaps a parent's response to a frightened child, becoming generalised into the reaching-out relationship to any fellow-being in trouble. As Peter Lomas remarked in this context: 'We would not classify him, nor take up an attitude of dispassionate scientific interest.'

In making this point, I by no means imply that professionalism has no value in my eyes. True, one does not have to be a professional to care. But the profession does introduce another dimension. It carries the assurance of competence and informed responsibility. My point is that professional knowledge, skill and experience, possessed and built upon, has to relate meaningfully to what the practice of caring is all about, namely the person. Professional skill should help us to perceive his *real* needs, and help us to a closer grasp of his actual experience. It should help to free us from concepts, philosophies and theories that would objectify him and fit him into categories, or direct him to what our prejudice would dictate he 'should' be. Professionalism should help us to know how we can participate in his situation with the knowledge and understanding we possess, so as to meet him in his anguish with help in our hands. It should help us to give him the relationship of insight and acceptance that he particularly needs in order to grow and become whole.

Approached in this way, I see no reason why our various professional attitudes as caring people should not tend towards a common understanding, the abolition of jargon (in thought as well as in word) and the beginning of a true language of the person.

The person in relationship

In talking about being a person and knowing a person, one refers to different aspects of the same thing, namely one's *personal relationship* with another person or persons to whom one is attached. One can only become, and continue to be, a person through relationship with another. In Martin Buber's language one speaks the word 'I–Thou', whereupon the speaker 'enters the word and takes his stand in it…' He takes his stand in *relation*. This is a basic primary truth about humans which is irreducible. It starts from the fact that when a baby is born it is separated from its mother in a personally helpless state – a potentially destructive position that is redeemed only because relationship is possible. It is only through the continuing relationship with mother that the baby can survive and grow. This is true of his whole self, not just his body. And the self can grow and develop towards autonomy only if the relationship is good enough to meet his need; and it is important to realise that this involves the need to experience *identification with another human being*, and is not merely a need for servicing. (Note – Parents do not have to be perfect!) The infant then continues to grow *as a person*. Unfortunately, however, not all experience is good enough. Events can, and do, occur within the baby's basic relationships that disturb him to a degree that exceeds his capacity to cope: hurt, separation, rejection, overpossessiveness, for example, which he cannot assimilate and lacks the resources to change. This causes a hold-up in his development. The baby's continuity as a developing person is interrupted. But he cannot stop the world until the problem is sorted out and normality restored. He has somehow to struggle with the bad, unacceptable manifestation of mother, while life with his 'real' mother goes on from day to day around him. The human infant resolves this problem by taking the 'bad' into himself. He then grapples with it in his inner world, while the daily life that he cannot alter goes on outside him. In his inner world, the personal reality of his needs and strivings is paramount. He has not yet learned how to objectify reality, much less to think logically. In grappling with the bad relationship (i.e. the bad aspect of a relationship) he tries to make it 'good', as well as trying to cope with his feelings about its badness. He forms an inner psychic representation of what he needs to happen (no longer taken for granted) and also of what he now expects to happen. This leaves him with a more or less serious problem that greatly affects his ability to relate to people from then on. As a growing person, he will have to continue to struggle with this, and other like problems, *within his own mind*; and these act as points of inhibited or distorted growth in his personality. Thus he will experience what began as a problem in relationship as having now become a personal problem within himself. And because who he is determines how he relates to other persons, he will find himself becoming involved emotionally with other people in a special way that reflects this inner problem – itself usually forgotten by this time, because it was split off in the past from the mainstream of everyday consciousness. It is as if, without realising it, he were constructing a relationship in which he could try again for a solution: a new relationship through which the inner sense that something is badly wrong could be resolved. Alas, this is usually a disappointing failure: the other person is uncomprehending and feels misunderstood, since he has, so to speak, a different script. This situation commonly underlies marriages that go wrong, and much unhappiness in families. It also provides the optimistic starting-point for counselling and psychotherapy, because our help is usually sought for just such problems in adult relationship, or by people who have become aware that something is badly wrong inside the self. It is to be hoped that we can unravel the underlying script.

I have put forward the view that underlying these problems is an interruption of the natural tendency to grow and develop as a person – a tendency that is inherent in human beings, and is the source of our therapeutic hope. We can see our task as caring persons as a skilled attempt to remove the obstacles, e.g. of mistrust, fear, anger or guilt, that inhibit the natural growth and being of the person; and we do this in so far as we succeed in being persons ourselves, capable of providing the right relationship needed to renew development towards wholeness and maturity.

The client and the professional are persons seeking each other. The former is attempting to create the relationship he needs; the latter perceives what is happening and provides what had been missing in the past – namely the necessary understanding, caring and support; and perhaps above all, recognition of the self in its uniqueness and value.

So often we see a caring response to a troubled person being obscured, or held back – becoming a relatively impersonal reaction to the person's *behaviour*, or directed to the front he represents, to which the carer can respond in a more or less standard way, perhaps as a result of certain professional training. This tends to maintain the front, or even to depersonalise the individual cared for; and it contrasts with a response which is the outcome of *joining in his experience*, which validates the person.

How far are our responses the outcome of entering into the experience of the other? How far are they merely a 'professional' reaction to behaviour as we interpret it? The difference seems crucial. Only a response based on one's ability to share in the other's experience can be really caring, really creative and liberating.

References:

Buber, Martin (1923) translated into English 1937: second (revised) edition 1959 'I and Thou.'
Laing, R D (1967) 'The Politics of Experience'
Lomas, Peter (1973) 'True and False Experience.'
Sutherland, J D (Malcolm Miller Lecture, 1979) 'The Psychodynamic Image of Man'

Some Thoughts about Training Counsellors

The best counsellors are not produced by training. They are *found*. The right kind of personality cannot be created by instruction. Wisdom, empathy and genuine caring cannot be inculcated by training procedures. One has to begin with a competent personality; and further development of competence comes from absorbing the rich experience of more senior counsellors who are themselves competent personalities, and particularly from work with the client, when it accompanies the development of the client's experience. This is the real 'continued professional development', and is more profound than a learned skill. The best learning comes not from instruction but from the support, understanding and encouragement of a more experienced person, known, trusted and liked by the counsellor. The worst learning comes from didactic instruction that buries the personality of the developing counsellor under the cloak of somebody else's (possibly dubious) ideas, to his great loss. Even self-conscious 'facilitation' is suspect, as it can so easily result in being led into somebody else's ways rather than to the discovery of one's own. The 'training analysis' of psychoanalysts seems to be a better training model, in that it puts the trainee through the same experiential process as the client – but that is far removed from the production-line of counsellors.

I think a lot more emphasis should be put on what the counselling process really is, rather than on what the practitioner should do. The whole essence of it lies in the authentic response of two people, each to the other, so that essential truths can be expressed openly; and this is possible only in an atmosphere of security and acceptance, where each values the other. Not everybody can bring this about, even with all the training available, and much effort and a plethora of words and high-sounding ideas cannot create this ability if the potential is not there to start with. I suspect that this awful truth is often concealed under the uneasy self-preoccupations and political manoeuvrings of counselling organisations and associations. It is not too difficult to produce impressive and high-sounding journals, papers, directives and so on. But what do these really do to the unconfident would-be counsellor except to reassure him that it is great to be involved in such a wonderful institution, and to leave him to make what he can of its seductive ideas? He will attend lectures, eager to be told what to do and what to think – how to restructure his natural self. And he has to pay handsomely for this experience.

You can teach somebody about painting or poetry or music, but you cannot *make* a creative artist by training alone. You can only help him to discover to what extent he is one or not. Counselling would seem to me to be a similar case. It is an ability that will emerge in a person so gifted – and not a few people are, fortunately – when it can be helped to emerge, but it cannot be put there by training if the gift is not there. We are talking about a process of discovery; and perhaps the emphasis should be on this concept in the work of the institutions and associations that take the responsibility for 'producing' counsellors. A deal of trouble and confusion might then be averted. In connection with this, some effort has surely also to be made, through selection, to identify those people who are actually looking for instruction and help because of insecurities in their own personalities. It is a serious matter when a counsellor purporting to help clients is in fact covertly seeking help for his own unacknowledged problems. And if he gets into the training hierarchy the result could be deadly.

Seminars and personal discussions can be helpful if the clear aim is to share experience, and thereby enrich the resources of insight and understanding. The mere imparting of knowledge can never be enough, and at worst could mislead. Words like 'technique' have a mechanistic connotation and are misleading, as they imply manipulating people in a particular way. A counsellor should not be 'doing something to' a person he is counselling. He should surely be helping that person to understand more profoundly what is going on within his own self in relation to others, by whatever means may be most appropriate in the particular case. We should be looking at how appropriate 'training' (another mechanistic word) might be helpful towards this end.

The process of training should follow closely the process of 'treating'. Neither is simply a process of telling someone what to do, or how to think. Like treating, counsellor training should promote *understanding*, not obedience to rules and precepts. For counsellors, all treating is training, and the schools should make this as conscious as possible.

The essential faculties at the heart of these processes are *insight* and *empathy*: insight into one's own mind and heart, and empathic insight into the heart and mind of the other person. These faculties must be consciously identified and nurtured, for upon them depends the success or failure of counselling training and practice. Identified and nurtured – they cannot be inculcated.

One of the worst, and most insidious, faults in counselling practice is the tendency alluded to above, namely to import one's own problems unconsciously into the situation, and mix them up with the client's problems. The apparent treatment of the client can then become a covert treatment of the counsellor. This intrusion of projective identification then binds counsellor and client in an unrecognised and unhealthy way – a mutually dependent bind – that spells the end of successful treatment. Training should therefore involve an assessment of the trainee's awareness of his own unresolved emotional difficulties. This problem requires great vigilance on the part of supervisors. It would not be enough merely to tell the trainee to beware of such risks. The problem is an unconscious one, which the conscious didactic approach cannot reach. Once again the emphasis is on the psychological state of the counsellor, not his or her learned skills. The training needed is the same basic process as counselling itself. Let him discover what his problems are, through relationship with his teacher. These are the problems that would cause difficulties with his subsequent clients were they to remain unconscious. And this process should continue throughout all his future practice in relationship with his supervisor.

I have stressed the weaknesses of a didactic 'school-masterish' type of training method. If a trainee is taught in this way he will tend to adopt the same method in his counselling – the pupil imitates the master, who can come to represent the 'right way to do it'. The client is then taught how to behave – which is to say that he acquires a superficial overlay that merely conceals his problems instead of helping to resolve them.

Much has been said and written about 'methods' and 'techniques'; but it has been found that the results of psychotherapy depend more upon the quality of the relationship between therapist and client than upon any particular technical method. I for one believe this to be profoundly true. The model of a good personal relationship has to be at the heart of the process of helping a person to form good personal relationships – which is what counselling is chiefly about. The counsellor passes on to the client what he has experienced in training. It is to be hoped that this is always fully recognised.

APPENDIX

What is Going Wrong?

I am concerned about the prevalence of social unrest in our society, particularly among young people, and I would like to write some notes in an attempt to understand it.

There is a tendency these days for physical sexual relationship among young people to become 'normalised'. This accompanies an increasing emphasis placed on sexuality in ever-extending aspects of life. Attractive objects are described as 'sexy'. Even Government documents are being 'sexed up'. Provocative images are everywhere. Older children cannot escape this influence, and are often unable to handle it in a balanced way. They are encouraged to learn about 'safe sex' before they have been able to grasp the realities of loving relationship. Contraceptives are readily available to them. Inevitably younger children are drawn in, and are influenced either thoughtlessly or deliberately by the entertainment industry and advertising. In such cases a balanced understanding cannot be expected, and damaging confusion can result. This imposes a huge responsibility upon those adults who have the care of small children entrusted to them, to keep sex in its rightful place. I fear that many of those adults have themselves been affected in early life by the adverse influences to which I have referred, and this problem should be recognised. It has deep roots and serious consequences. Emotionally damaged children make inadequate parents or carers, who in turn pass the problem on, and a chain of pathology is established. In the case of schoolchildren, abstinence is often not advocated as normal behaviour. Children should surely be led to believe that they do not have to *act* on the sexual feelings they have, but this is not always done. On the contrary, to the youngster virginity can be a sign of low standing among peers, and one is led to assume that this state of affairs is not questioned, if not actually approved of, by the adults in charge.

These issues are part of a wider change in our culture that has accelerated from the post-war period of social 'liberation'. There has been a weakening of family bonds, and changes in the interpretation of parental responsibility. There has arisen a clear choice between personal 'freedom' to do what one wants to satisfy personal ambition (e.g. in lifestyle and career), and the responsibilities of parenthood. On the one hand, both women and men direct their energies into activities that are only indirectly (if at all) related to the emotional needs of their children, and on the other hand there is the view that if you have children they should come first. If, as so often happens, personal choices come first, the children tend to become something to be coped with – handed over to other available adults or professional child-minders, so as not to interfere with what has become the 'real' business of life. The older institution of the Public School has remained for those who can afford it. So instead of being supported in expressing his real anxieties, the infant, toddler or early adolescent is made to suppress these feelings as best he can. His emotional needs are overlooked, denied, scoffed at or argued away – potentially with serious consequences. A child cannot become a secure and confident complete person without experiencing these attributes through a close and loving contact with adults who are themselves secure and confident in relation to him or her. In this relationship the child absorbs as his own the quality of a parental attitude to him. How else can respect for others arise in a child? He cannot grow up in an emotional desert. He grows through relationship. These qualities develop within him from his experience of loving respect and security within a nurturing attachment, which puts him first in the meeting of his real needs. It must be noted that this relationship is established uniquely with the primary carer – ideally the natural mother. A child cannot benefit emotionally if he is shuttled around between different carers. He is merely bewildered by this, and at a deep level insecure, no matter how genuinely dedicated the other carers are. I sometimes think that some people understand this more with their pets than with their children!

If such a unique maternal relationship is not adequately provided, the child is to that extent deprived – handicapped in trying to become a whole human being, lacking adequate emotional food, and therefore unable to grow as he should. This opens the way to many personal and social problems, and many children find themselves on this problematic route. It can take different forms according to circumstances, but inadequate relationship lies at the root of it. Currently a problem of obesity is recognised. Children are eating excessively (often junk food) as a substitute for missing emotional sustenance, and there are many other behavioural and health problems arising from that source.

If a child has not grown up in real relationship of the kind described, he or she has no inner sense of security with others. He cannot sense 'goodness' in them because he has no root experience of goodness, and cannot feel it, however much he may believe in it or intellectually grasp that there must be such a thing. A secure child carries within himself the awareness of being a proper person, through having been treated as a proper person, so incorporating essentially good values from the good parent who nurtured him. If this has not happened, the feeling of being 'good' is lacking – despite anything he may be taught through his rational mind. Here we are not dealing with thinking or logic, but the deeper belief of feeling. I am alarmed at the increase in numbers of children diagnosed as suffering from Asperger's syndrome.

What are the consequences of this deprivation? They will come from the young person's attempts to build a life for himself, by trying to find some way of coping with the vacuum. He has to try to find elsewhere an emotional satisfaction that will give his life some sense of meaning. His social environment offers many and varied possibilities, some of which we have mentioned above; and because whatever the resulting substitute behaviour is, it deals with a deep and very basic need that tends to feel essential and to become addictive. Of course many emotionally handicapped children fortunately do find ways that are socially acceptable if not wholly adequate; but the less fortunate get carried away all too easily by a prevailing culture which is anything but desirable. Sexual behaviour is an obvious way to seek emotional satisfaction, and the provocative stimuli are all around; but because in this context it is not associated with a real loving relationship, it is perpetually unsatisfying – so the search becomes promiscuous, and leads to addiction. Highly available alcohol is another common false substitute for an absent comforting attachment – again addictive, emotionally as well as physically – and drug addiction comes into the same category. Apart from these, we find all kinds of social misbehaviour among young people resulting from the fact that they cannot find a substitute for a missing relationship that gives them any peace. They go about angry with the world. In their hearts they are angry babies whose mother never satisfied them. We can see the obvious connection here with crime. Such emotional states can very easily result in robbery and violence, crimes of envy and jealousy and much other antisocial behaviour.

Another relevant issue in the forefront today is obesity, which has acquired the status of a disease, to be fought with drugs and/or diet and exercise. No doubt faulty diet and overeating are involved, but the important thing to look at is the cause of this behaviour, rather than to impose instructions and conditions that can be resisted or disregarded. Perhaps we should look at the problem in the light of what I have said already about addiction, and the underlying importance of faulty relationship in the individual's background. Perhaps the higher incidence of obesity among the underprivileged is not solely due to junk food, but also, and perhaps primarily, to disturbed relationships in an overstressed and anxious community – a serious social problem.

Now there is the much publicised 'yob culture', which is frequently associated with binge drinking. This has been taken seriously by the Government, and through this the police have been involved specifically to deal with antisocial behaviour – implying that it is something to be deterred by punishment, control and public humiliation. This approach would seem to me to provoke bitter resentment and further aggressive behaviour. What else could we expect? I believe it would be more effective to examine the causes of aggressive behaviour – in other words to regard it as another manifestation of failed relationships between the offenders and the rest of society. They are behaving like neglected or unwanted children, who will clearly not be 'cured' by further rejection. I cannot be drawn into proposing a cure aimed at the offenders. That is a political question. But I think that it should be based upon the right premises. The real problem is the parents, and other adults responsible for their upbringing, from whom the children have no option but to learn how to behave.

I would repeat that a very great deal of social unrest has its origin in the absence or loss of necessary nurturing relationship during infancy, carried on throughout childhood and adolescence, when the basic experiences needed for secure personality growth are laid down. An unfulfilling (and therefore hopeless) substitute is then sought at a time that is too late developmentally for reparation, and the substitute sources that offer themselves tend to exploit the tragedy for financial gain. Only a really secure caring relationship over time might help to make things more tolerable, but because in the adolescent it is occurring at a time too late to be properly internalised, such a relationship would need to be permanent – or rupture would then be a disaster.

The problem of what can be done is certainly formidable, but the first step has to be a general understanding of what it is. Here I have proposed a psychological theory, based upon what is known about the psychopathology of human development. The concepts of such theory, dare I say, may themselves have been modified these days by the prevailing culture – and, I suspect, may now follow less personal, more materialistic concepts that match the current social norms. Of course there must be other views on other premises. But what is needed at the moment is a serious interest, and serious discussion, involving as many sources as possible. This would surely be a hopeful starting point.

Where do we find the other premises? One that overlaps the above is that of morality and spiritual values. A new person is born into the world physically from the mother, with whom he remains an extension as it were, throughout his infancy. Later he becomes autonomous through the development of his genetic capabilities. But he is also a being endowed with life, with all its potentialities and values; and these assert themselves progressively as autonomy increases, leading to the necessity for his making choices. He is a descendant of Adam, and carries the potentialities of both good and evil in his nature. Therein a struggle could arise between self-will and what he discovers of moral good. But this discovery is not necessarily the imposed rules of adults. There can also be an appeal to an inner sense of what later comes to be felt as goodness – a moral value. The tendency these days is to look on moral values epistemologically, as knowledge acquired by learning, rather than existentially, as a given quality in the human soul. These concepts are matters of opinion, but the choice is important. If goodness is learned, morality would appear to be dependent on the custom of the age, although here a consistent attitude to religion could play a part, pointing to an existential component. In our country this latter attitude is waning, and with it an acceptance of the spiritual value of the human person. So the choice between right and wrong is reduced to a matter of obedience or disobedience to human authority: 'Everybody can be good if they want to be. If they don't, they must be coerced into changing their ways.' There is little if any recognition of an inner knowledge of goodness that has been blocked, but which can be freed by kind and caring relationship. Is it not so that all persons were innocent once? What have we done to them? Perhaps we have to go back in time to find out.

If a child has to be taught what is good and what is bad, it implies that his mind is, morally, a blank slate. My contention is that if he has *experienced* an early loving relationship with another person he has, in his being, an awareness of the reality of 'goodness' which he does not owe to didactic moral teaching. And he feels 'badness' as an infringement of his natural state, which enters consciousness as unease or distress. Experience within that state can be the basis for discovering the moral values of right and wrong, by building up an understanding of these matters in line with the deeper understanding that is already there. This contrasts with the didactic practice that stamps these values as foreign concepts upon a child who may lack the inner assimilated experience to enable proper acceptance and true understanding. Such a child may go on to seek ways of circumventing these learned principles and simply do what he wants, through lack of the deep inner feeling of rightness – from which such behaviour could not arise.

This consideration leads naturally to the topic of guilt. Freud's idea of a superego derived from a dominant father is clearly based on the 'blank slate' idea of moral behaviour, which some might call materialistic, or even atheistic. It presumes no pre-existing source which can be contacted by loving experience. Freud's concept of the inner self was a raging force demanding gratification, which he appropriately called the 'Id' (literally the Thing). This force was hammered into the shape demanded by social culture by the child's domineering father, internalised as what he called the 'Super-ego' (something superior to the self). The force exerted by the Super-ego on the Id gives rise to guilt – for wanting an inbred satisfaction that was forbidden. In this scheme Good is simply the absence of Bad, and seems to have no other basis. This view would seem to be primitive in the extreme, missing out what seems to me to be the essential core of humanity. In a sense, morality has disappeared in a system of domination and guilt, in which the person has no moral choice – simply obedience, to avoid pain. It may be that Freud's ideas arose from the concept of the Jewish God, with whom goodness arose from obedience and sacrifice. To continue the theological argument further, one can compare the ancient Hebrew scheme with the vastly different teaching of the New Testament, where the Christian doctrine that God is Love is consistent with the developmental ideas propounded above about the origin in love of goodness and right behaviour.

I have heard it said that a child nurtured to be secure and happy will consider himself to be the centre of the earth, and treat others with disdain. This is nonsense. That child will treat the other in accordance with his internalised image as an equal in mutually caring relationship. Alas, he may find out later, to his sorrow, that in the world at large very different responses have to be experienced and adapted to, because there exist in the world powerful and disturbing influences that would appear to arise from a very basic prevalence of the 'unloved' state (to use the above terminology) in humanity as a whole. The exercise of power and coercion, either brutally, or under the guise of altruism, by governments and individuals, has percolated throughout human life from time immemorial. It is as if the world at large were behaving like an insecure unloved child – and as if civilisation were an attempt to seek another way to find peace. Not a very satisfactory way, as history shows. I seem to deduce from this that the mass of humanity feels exiled from a loving relationship that alone would bring peace. The gates of Eden have closed behind it.

This inference draws the mind inexorably to a theological premise. We appear to be talking about humanity's alienation from God, and this in turn introduces the topic of original sin, since the absolute love of God is constant by definition. 'Man's first disobedience...' begins *Paradise Lost*. Psychologists have considered this as a metaphor for the child's transition from the innocence of infancy to the self-conscious choices facing the early adolescent in his emergent independence – no longer subject entirely to the adults' will, but faced with responsibility for his own life, errors of judgement and all. This is a tempting analogy. The sticking-point is the conception of *sin*, with the implication that growing up is evil. Ancient Judaism did regard sexuality, the hallmark of puberty, as impure, and surrounded it with strict prohibitions as if it were sinful, and this tendency has remained in the Christian tradition. As a result, much emotional disturbance and neurosis has arisen, and the modern emphasis has moved somewhat away from sin to pathology. But a degree of prohibition has remained, although seen now as arising from wrongs of hygiene rather than immorality. It is this situation that has now brought about a virtual removal of prohibition. But the pendulum has swung too far, and I have been pleading for a return to continence as a *normal* condition of loving care prevailing in growing up, that would entail health and hygiene as a consequence.

I must return to my conviction that it is on the health of *relationship* between persons that the physical, emotional and moral health of individuals and of society, and of the human race as a whole, depends. And healthy relationship begins in the family, between parents and child. This is arguably the most important thing in life, and we have been allowing it to become sidelined. This, I think, is what has gone wrong.

24 November 2004

This essay was included in 'Carl and other writings' by Mirabelle Maslin, 2005

Ten Years After

'How mad do we have to get before sanity sets in?
When does the night of cruelty end and the morning of compassion
begin? When does civilisation start?'
Colin Simpson, in 'Picture of Japan.'

What has happened to civilisation in our country since the war? Crimes of violence have gone up, drug addiction has gone up, mental instability, divorce, immorality of all kinds – what evil has not soared? The cost of living, hours of work and the difficulties of survival for many, are, if anything, more unequal now than were their pre-war precursors. This is surely the decline of civilised life. Our age is passing into ruin. Everywhere the gutted edifice of our culture is tottering, despite expedient props. We live in anxiety, awaiting an impending crash. There are virtually no places in which to relax in peace, no sanctuary from noise and clutter. The battered shell in which we live is overcrowded and barren. True, there are some who have dug out a more pleasant place for themselves and appear to be content; but they would be nonetheless vulnerable if the crash should come. They only imagine that they are better off. Many who have known the pleasures and elegance of what this structure once was, those who have struggled to achieve its betterment, haunt its broken and blackened walls, silently, and with frightened eyes. What purpose have they now, without security, without enthusiasm, without hope? They try to save themselves; but their destiny is to witness the degeneracy of their generation all around them; to watch and mourn the corruption of children; to stand helpless, while a mantle of spiritual death envelops them one by one. They lose in the end always, even although their livelihood is not denied them, because it is beyond mortal power to give direction and purpose to those who do not know they need it. Only, perhaps, when it is too late, they will wake up and search for their lost lives, crying across the waste of years for what once might have been. But by then it is too late. Time cannot be reversed to give them a second chance. So they are left alone, those who have defended themselves against the struggling realities of life, to face it with the only thing they ever prized or sought – their own pitiable selves!

Those who cannot *feel* love and care for others, in spite of what they may believe, nourish in their hearts the only truly basic evil in the world, from which all others spring. They tend to see life as behaviour to be practised according to a book of etiquette, as it were; but they spread suffering and spiritual death among those others who need real caring. May God pity their children. These are the loveless ones, who live with no real caring, and form the next generation of the lost. These little ones do not know that there is any other life. They cannot know what they have never experienced. Nor can they help being endlessly dependent, because their needs are never satisfied. They survive like objects, kept going by food and water, or the precursor of such fuel, namely money. In the depths of their hearts there is at first an instinctual awareness that there must be somebody to care for them, so that they may live; and because of the inadequacy of such care, there arises anxiety, pain and sorrow that may never leave them. They cannot respond to the mechanical facts of money being spent on them. The feeling can arise that they are an expensive nuisance. Yet often the parents bid each other up, to show how much they 'care' for their children. And from the children they expect interest to be paid in the form of gratitude and reflected credit, 'See what I did for you!'... 'If it hadn't been for me!' ... So they sneer, as if to remind the wretched child that God and man would turn against him for failing to fall down and worship. So he devotes his ruined life to paying his debt for the privilege of having been born. Such children never become true individuals, but either remain mere family possessions or investments, or become social outcasts.

Of course there are many who rebel; but most of these have brief, desperate careers that are quickly crushed, because in the eyes of the world they are wrong. They bruise their fists against the stone wall of a society which will not let them in. Wherever they go they are shunned as examples of bad temper, selfishness and ingratitude. Understandably, they usually end up by losing all faith in everything, believing in nothing but their own wits and the strength of their hands. They become reckless, undisciplined and criminal because they don't care any more. Why should they, when nobody cared for them? After all, that is what they have learned. And even yet, nobody ever knows how empty, how desperately lonely they are inside. Instead, the law-abiding citizen hits them back, and glows with self-righteousness when they are locked up, as they often are, in prison.

When will people realise that the only real sin is self-love, which cannot give warmth and life to a child? When will they discover that the only truly unbearable suffering is the loneliness of being unwanted and unloved? When will the day come when the truth will be known that perfect love casteth out fear, and the noblest virtue is the giving of love for sheer joy, without thought of self?

One may think it strange that people say they know this, and really believe in their Christianity, yet in practice are so cruel and cause so much misery. It is a curious fact that human beings have the unfortunate power to blind themselves to what they do not wish to see! I am afraid we all harbour quite inaccurate illusions about ourselves. The greatest cruelty has been practised in the name of God. Holiness, virtue and liberty have been the banners of those who hate their fellow men. The most dangerous tyrant is he who feels no mercy or remorse because his cruelty is sanctified by a religious belief, which he equates with moral law. Then he can invoke the will of God. His victims cannot rebel without damning themselves further. Hence the horrors of the Crusades, the Holy Inquisition, the French Revolution, the seventeenth-century religious strife in Britain and much else. Even Ezra

Pound, who was no advocate of social freedom, denounced the moral stranglehold of sanctimonious piety as 'the tyranny of the unimaginative'.

The common man is unimaginative, it seems. One can scarcely believe how ignorant he is of himself and others. He thinks he is good and kind when he is merely bigoted and selfish. He thinks he loves his girl when he is merely flattered by her attention. He thinks he is helping his fellows when he is merely making use of them. He thinks that friends are people who agree with everything he says, while those who differ from him are enemies. He is the common criminal who can be condemned and sentenced by others as bigoted and as self-assured as himself. Is he not you and I? All of us?

1956

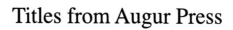

Titles from Augur Press

Poems of Wartime Years

ISBN 978-0-9549551-6-8 £4.99

by W N Taylor

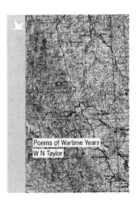

My experience of World War II was in the Far East - South East Asia Command (SEAC), but these are not 'war poems' in the ordinary sense.

They are thoughts and memories of the periphery rather than the centre of action, and reflections afterwards in subsequent years, some pertaining to other wars, bearing the stamp of futility, cynicism, sadness and a flicker of hope. I was a medical student when the war began in 1939, larking about with my friends, (see A Cycle of Sonnets) but knowing that when we qualified we would be called up. After serving with an infantry battalion in coastal defence on the Isle of Wight, I was posted to a West African division and accompanied them into the jungles of Burma. This involved a fight against disease as well as the Japanese. When this was over, I sailed off with my African soldiers and returned them to their homes in the Gold Coast, now called Ghana.

Order from your local bookshop, amazon.co.uk or
the Augur Press website at www.augurpress.com

Infants and Children
An introduction to emotional development

ISBN 978-0-9571380-2-5   £7.99

by Mirabelle Maslin

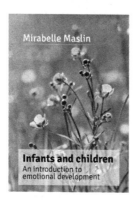

A parent's ability to be able to see and understand things through the eyes of their child is fundamental. The child will come to feel truly known by the parent, and the parent helps him to make sense of what surrounds him.

Where can true comfort be found? True comfort arises from the knowledge of relationship that is based on trust.

And what about the needs of the child of the past that dwells inside each 'adult' state?

This book opens up a whole new world of understanding for parents and carers.

Order from your local bookshop, amazon.co.uk or the Augur Press website at www.augurpress.com

Titles from Augur Press

Self-help novellas
  by Mirabelle Maslin
Miranda   £6.99   978-0-9558936-5-0
Lynne   £6.99   978-0-9558936-6-7
Field Fare   £6.99   978-0-9558936-8-1

Poetry
The Poetry Catchers   £7.99   978-0-9549551-9-9
  by Pupils from Craigton Primary
  School
Poems of Wartime Years   £4.99   978-0-9549551-6-8
  by W N Taylor
The Voice Within   £5.99   978-0-9558936-3-6
  by Catherine Turvey
Now Is Where We Are   £6.99   978-0-9558936-7-4
  by Hilary Lissenden

Trilogy by Mirabelle Maslin
Beyond the Veil   £8.99   978-0-9549551-4-4
Fay   £8.99   978-0-9549551-3-7
Emily   £8.99   978-0-9549551-8-2

Other novels
One Eye Open: Can a Dolphin   £7.99   978-0-9571380-1-8
Save the World?
  by Steve Cameron
The Candle Flame   £7.99   978-0-9558936-1-2
  by Mirabelle Maslin
Letters to my Paper Lover   £7.99   978-0-9549551-1-3
  by Fleur Soignon

For children and young people
The Supply Teacher's Surprise   £5.99   978-0-9558936-4-3
  by Mirabelle Maslin
Tracy by Mirabelle Maslin   £6.95   978-0-9549551-0-6
The Fifth Key   £7.99   978-0-9558936-0-5
  by Mirabelle Maslin

Child development
Infants and children: £7.99   978-0-9571380-2-5
emotional development

Eating disorder
Size Zero and Beyond: £13.99   978-0-9571380-0-1
A personal study of anorexia
nervosa by Jacqueline M Kemp

Hemiplegia
Hemiplegic Utopia: Manc Style   £6.99   978-0-9549551-7-5
  by Lee Seymour

Sexual Abuse
Carl and other writings   £5.99   978-0-9549551-2-0
  by Mirabelle Maslin

Health
Mercury in Dental Fillings   £5.99   978-0-9558936-2-9
  by Stewart J Wright
Lentigo Maligna Melanoma: £5.99   978-0-9558936-9-8
A sufferer's tale
  by Mirabelle Maslin

Miscellaneous
On a Dog Lead   £6.99   978-0-9549551-5-1
  by Mirabelle Maslin

Ordering online   **www.augurpress.com**

By Post   Delf House, 52, Penicuik Road, Roslin,
      Midlothian EH25 9LH UK

Postage and packing: £2.00 for each book, and add £0.75p for each
additional item. Cheques payable to Augur Press.

Prices and availability subject to change without notice. When placing your
order, please indicate if you do not wish to receive any additional information.

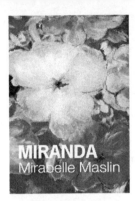
MIRANDA
Mirabelle Maslin

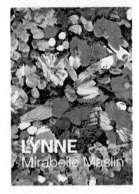
LYNNE
Mirabelle Maslin

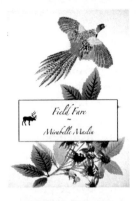
Field Fare
~
Mirabelle Maslin

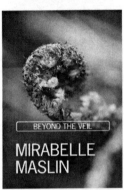
BEYOND THE VEIL
MIRABELLE
MASLIN

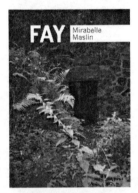
FAY Mirabelle
Maslin

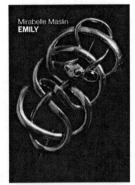
Mirabelle Maslin
EMILY

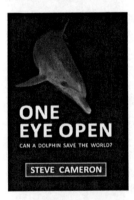
ONE
EYE OPEN
CAN A DOLPHIN SAVE THE WORLD?
STEVE CAMERON

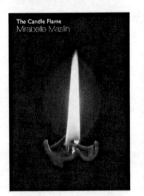
The Candle Flame
Mirabelle Maslin

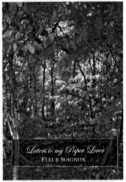
Letters to my Paper Lover
FLEUR SOIGNON

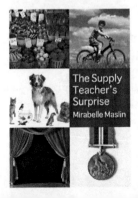
The Supply
Teacher's
Surprise
Mirabelle Maslin

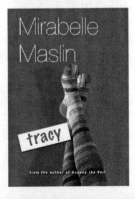
Mirabelle
Maslin
tracy
from the author of Beyond the Veil

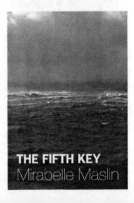
THE FIFTH KEY
Mirabelle Maslin

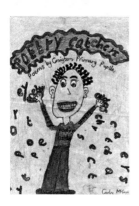

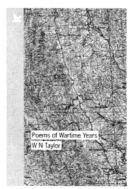

Poems of Wartime Years
W N Taylor

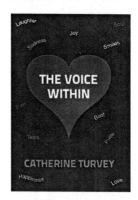

THE VOICE
WITHIN

CATHERINE TURVEY

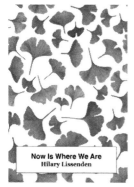

Now Is Where We Are
Hilary Lissenden

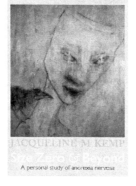

JACQUELINE M KEMP
Size Zero & Beyond
A personal study of anorexia nervosa

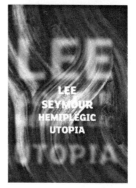

LEE
SEYMOUR
HEMIPLEGIC
UTOPIA

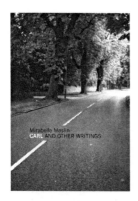

Mirabelle Maslin
CARL AND OTHER WRITINGS

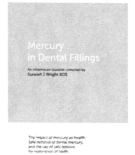

Mercury
in Dental Fillings

An information booklet compiled by
Stewart J Wright BDS

The impact of mercury on health.
Safe removal of dental mercury,
and the use of safe options
for restoration of teeth.

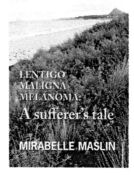

LENTIGO
MALIGNA
MELANOMA:
A sufferer's tale

MIRABELLE MASLIN

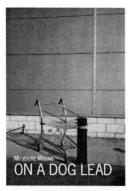

Mirabelle Maslin
ON A DOG LEAD

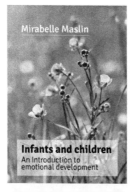

Mirabelle Maslin

Infants and children
An introduction to
emotional development

Lightning Source UK Ltd.
Milton Keynes UK
UKOW05f1356250414

230578UK00007B/74/P